Principles of Surgical Technique

The Art of Surgery

Second Edition

Principles of Surgical Technique

The Art of Surgery

Second Edition

by

Gary G. Wind, MD, FACS
Associate Professor of Surgery
Assistant Professor of Anatomy
Uniformed Services University of the Health Sciences
Bethesda, Maryland

Norman M. Rich, MD, FACS
Professor and Chairman
Department of Surgery
Uniformed Services University of the Health Sciences
Bethesda, Maryland

With contributions by ALAN E. SEYFER, M.D and DAVID M. LICHTMAN, M.D.

Illustrated by GARY G. WIND, M.D.

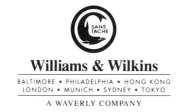

Williams & Wilkins

BALTIMORE • PHILADELPHIA • HONG KONG
LONDON • MUNICH • SYDNEY • TOKYO

A WAVERLY COMPANY

Editor: Charles W. Mitchell
Copy Editor: Starr Belsky
Designer: Gary Wind, Linda Powell

Copyright © Gary Wind, Urban & Schwarzenberg 1987
Williams & Wilkins
428 East Preston Street
Baltimore, Maryland 21202, USA

Accurate indications, adverse reactions, and dosage schedules for drugs are provided in this book, but it is possible that they may change. The reader is urged to review the package information data of the manufacturers of the medications mentioned.

First Edition 1983

Library of Congress Cataloging in Publication Data

Wind, Gary G.
  Principles of surgical technique.

  Bibliography: p.
  Includes index.
  Surgery, Operative. I. Rich, Norman M. II. Title.
[DNLM: 1. Surgery, Operative. WO 500 W763 p]
RD32.W56 1986   617′.9   86-15910
ISBN 0-8067-2162-6

98 99
7 8 9 10

Dedication

To Merri, Rebecca, and David

Contents

Part I
Definition of the Principles

Part II
Application of the Principles

Foreword to the Second Edition

I was given the opportunity in 1983 of reviewing the first edition of this book for the *New England Journal of Medicine*. My review included the statement, "In this book the authors have succeeded in writing a book on surgery in a truly original manner. This is a difficult feat, rarely achieved."

Many forewords are largely congratulatory. In this foreword I will criticize, in a constructive manner I hope, and then praise and congratulate as I did in 1983. The second edition of this book is even better than the first. The historical section has been expanded and improved, Alan Seyfer has provided a major addition to the chapter on wound healing, surgical staplers now rate a full chapter, and David Lichtman has covered microsurgery in an outstanding way. There is an entirely new chapter, a "Surgical Anatomy of the Abdomen," which has been made necessary by the new information produced by computed tomography and magnetic resonance imaging. These techniques have given us a view of the anatomy of this region in the living human which was not available before. In this chapter, as in all the others, the superb illustrations drawn by Gary Wind add immensely to the text.

A major objective of this book is to teach third- and fourth-year medical students and junior surgical residents how to handle human tissues so that optimum wound healing will occur. The concept of packing in wound management is often erroneously interpreted by the novice. The word "packing" is defined in *Dorland's Illustrated Medical Dictionary* as "the act of filling a wound with gauze, sponges, pads or other materials." In my opinion it is common for wounds to be packed tightly, and the gauze or other material is literally rammed in. This can be very harmful. It is better to pack the wound very loosely. The word loosely should be placed after the word pack in every case.

I was interested to learn that Fioravante in 1570 urinated on the severed nose of the patient to cleanse it before he secured it back into position. We sometimes forget that in most people urine is a sterile fluid. In World War II it was widely used by German soldiers to extinguish fragments of phosphorous that were burning in their tissues; a buddy system was often employed. Fortunately for us, phosphorous was not available in sufficient quantities in Germany for it to be used against us as an ingredient in missiles of war.

Sutures of polypropylene, nylon, and other materials have been well tested and tried. It is my personal view that sutures of polytetrafluoroethylene will be found superior to both these materials and will be used increasingly. Advantages include a needle size that is the same size as the suture and the fact that the suture does not kink, coil, twist, and knot in the way a polypropylene suture does.

Again, I congratulate the authors on an excellent book that will be very valuable to senior medical students and junior residents.

CHARLES ROB, M. D.
Professor of Surgery
Uniformed Services University of the Health Sciences
F. Edward Hebert School of Medicine
Bethesda, Maryland

IX

Foreword to the First Edition

For most surgical patients, the most important thing that happens during their hospital stay is the surgical operation itself. If the patient enters with severe injury, it is the function of the surgical operation to abate the stress. To do this, the surgeon must avoid contamination and infection, immobilize fractures, exteriorize holed hollow viscera, reestablish normal ventilatory mechanics, relieve pressure in the brain, and drain abcesses, to give a few examples. This being done, the normal built-in processes of convalescence can begin their work.

If elective surgery is in store for the patient, then the surgeon's ideal is to carry out the anatomic and pathologic objectives of the procedure with the least distortion of the patient's homeostatic mechanism, with the least tissue injury.

Thus, while surgery in its very nature deals with tissue injury, it is in the one instance seeking to abate an injury imposed from the outside, and in the other, to minimize that necessarily imposed by the surgeon himself.

In either event, effective surgery results in a lesser load on the total organism. With surgical excellence there is a wound to heal with little dead space, detritus, or bacteria; homeostatic physiology less burdened by challenge of volume loss or the low flow state; minimal respiratory or biochemical distortion, coagulation difficulties, or excessive transfusion.

This book will find its most responsive audience amongst those beginning surgery. These might be young men and women in their third or fourth year of medical school who are starting to see surgical patients, talk with them, treat them, and assist at their operations. Or, the readers may be surgical interns starting out their careers, or junior residents. The authors discuss some of the most basic and deceptively simple things concerning the handling of soft tissues, of instruments, and of suture materials.

If a book such as this results in a smoother convalescence, and a "lesser load" for patients after injury or elective surgery, it will have accomplished its purpose. If it helps a young person to enter this challenging and rewarding profession with a lesser feeling of insecurity and ignorance, it will have more than justified the price of time or resources spent in its composition acquisition, and persual.

Congratulations to the authors (one of them the artist, also) for producing a fine beginners' book on surgical techniques.

FRANCIS D. MOORE, M. D.
Moseley Professor of Surgery, Emeritus
Harvard Medical School

Surgeon-in-Chief, Emeritus
Peter Bent Brigham Hospital
Boston, Massachusetts

Preface

*"The young surgeon who learns the basic precepts of
asepsis, hemostasis, adequate exposure and gentleness
to tissue has mastered his most difficult lessons."*
ROBERT M. ZOLLINGER, 1975

Good surgery is based on a central set of interrelated principles that may be conveniently divided into groups related to the surgeon: asepsis, tissue handling, hemostasis, and exposure. The common overriding concern in all these is to do no harm. This book shows how basic principles are used to achieve that goal.

Many good surgical texts contain encyclopedic amounts of surgical knowledge. Surgical atlases describe detailed, step-by-step techniques for performing operations. Neither, however, presents a unified, logical explication of the basic principles that bridge the gap between "knowing" and "doing." At most one finds a paragraph or page devoted to "surgical technique" restating Halsted's contributions. This lack of attention does not represent negligence on the part of authors, for it is extremely difficult to communicate these principles on paper. Many surgical educators think that the abstract concepts relating to technique are best learned in the operating room.

However, there are several problems with learning solely by experience. Much surgical teaching occurs in a one-to-one setting, and not every surgeon is a good teacher. The exposure of residents to various surgical problems is not uniform even within a single institution, let alone from one place to another. The ratio of staff to residents often dictates that the attending surgeon scrub with the senior residents while the junior house staff are taught by the next higher resident. This too is a bad arrangement! The resident has the least exposure to those who can teach him good technique during the very time when he is expected to learn it. The rationalization that the junior resident will learn with experience is inconsistent with the assumption that the senior resident has acquired technical competence in the early stages of training.

The attention devoted to the junior residents varies with the quality of each surgical training program. Even in the best program, however, sloppy and erroneous technique can be passed on and incorporated into a developing surgeon's style. When the resident learns faulty technique, the patient suffers from the resident's mistakes, and the resident has a difficult time unlearning bad technique later. It is, therefore, important to present in one place an outline of the principles practiced by the best surgeons so that the resident can get an overview and recognize those areas in which his exposure has been limited.

The content of this book complements the didactic information found in texts and atlases and in no way diminishes the need to master that knowledge; rather, the book is an adjunct to its application. This book is about the principles of technique rather than techniques of performing specific operations themselves. Work-up, decision making, monitoring, and critical care are subjects found in surgical texts. The mechanical aspects of sterilization, scrubbing, gowning, gloving, positioning the patient, and draping are dealt with in technical manuals. The major concern of this book is what the surgeon does in the operating room.

This book is not intended or designed to teach surgery to nonsurgeons, but others besides junior surgical residents can benefit from a discussion of principles of surgical technique. Medical students may better appreciate the surgery they see if they are aware of these underlying concepts. Both operating room and floor nurses may gain a better understanding of the surgeon's concerns and actions if they know the rationale behind them. Senior house staff and attending staff may find the book useful as a teaching resource. Nonsurgeons should find the discussion enlightening.

The overwhelmingly favorable response to the first edition and the counsel of many distinguished educators encouraged us to expand on these themes in this second edition. The historical perspective has been extended from Roman times to the dawn of the modern surgical era to highlight the incredible hardships faced by surgeon and patient prior to antisepsis, antibiotics, and anesthesia. A new section dealing with the clinical aspects of surgical and traumatic wounds has been added to complement the physiology of wound healing. A new chapter deals with surgical stapling devices. Although the novice surgeon must first learn how to deal with tissues manually, staplers have become a generally accepted part of the surgical armamentarium and warrant at least an introduction early in training. An example of the use of the stapler has been added to the chapter on small-bowel anastomosis. A second new chapter introduces the relatively new discipline of microsurgery. Despite the fact that it is a highly technical field beyond the level of the basic technique presented in this book, its inclusion is legitimate and useful for two reasons. First, it embodies in microcosm all the principles this book endeavors to teach and demonstrates the universal applicability of those principles. Second, microsurgery cuts across the boundaries of virtually every surgical specialty, from neurosurgery in the head to orthopedics in the toe, and the surgical trainee will necessarily be exposed to it and may even have the opportunity to assist. Thus an early introduction is timely.

The chapter on surgical anatomy of the abdomen has been totally rewritten with all new illustrations, as has the section on inguinal anatomy. A new section dealing with surgical drains discusses the history, indications, contraindications, and management of abdominal and soft tissue drains. New material has also been added to the chapters on knots and suture material and on vascular anastomosis.

Surgery's reputation for rigorous exactitude has made "surgical precision" a catchphrase in the English language. The young surgeon will find that it takes some practice and effort to bring his surgical craftmanship to a level justifying that catchphrase.

Acknowledgments

We remain indebted to those who helped with the preparation of the first edition: Dr. John Sharefkin, Dr. Hynda Kleinman, Dr. Michael Sheridan, Dr. Geoffrey Graeber, Diane Abeloff, AMI, Nan Curtis Tyler, and John Cronin.

We appreciate the generous advice and support of the many distinguished surgical educators whose critique of the first edition guided us in preparing the second. We wish to thank those who lent their expert assistance to the preparation of this second edition: Dr. Robert Joy for his advice on historical highlights in the development of surgical technique; Dr. Alan Seyfer for writing the second half of the chapter on wound healing; Dr. Charles Rob for reviewing the chapter on staplers; Dr. David Lichtman for writing the chapter on microsurgery; Dr. Jim Gross for reviewing the new chapter on surgical anatomy of the abdomen; Dr. Daniel Abramson for his expert advice on presenting the subject of surgical drains; and Dr. Lionel Villavicencio for contributing to the chapter on vascular anastomosis.

And finally, we are grateful to our editor, Mr. Charles Mitchell, for encouraging us to prepare this new edition; both he and Mr. Norman Och provided expert help in putting it together.

"Chyrurgerie is an art, which teacheth the way by reason, how by the operation of the hand we may cure, prevent and mitigate diseases, which accidentally happen upon us."

AMBROISE PARÉ, 1582

Part I

Definition of the Principles

Introduction

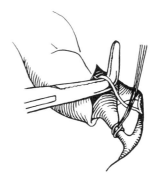

The Format

The book is divided into two parts. The first part outlines the broad fundamental principles of surgical technique. A historical perspective on the evolution of preanesthetic and preantiseptic surgical technique sets the stage. This is followed by a concise description of wound healing in relation to the technical principles of surgery. The next chapters – on knots, suture materials, instruments, and maneuvers – present the specific details of surgical technique, which are missing from most books on operative surgery. This is followed by discussions of the roles played by the surgical assistant and the operating-room team. The last two chapters in part I introduce two more advanced technical areas, staplers and microsurgery, that will be encountered by the surgical trainee and require some familiarity.

Part II is designed to illustrate by example the principles set out in part I. The first chapter discusses technique as it applies to several minor surgical procedures. The next chapter, "Surgical Anatomy of the Abdomen," digresses briefly to present some important clinical relationships within the abdominal cavity as background for the remaining chapters. The exemplary procedures that follow are common surgical operations in order of increasing complexity. In most cases a single method is shown so as not to distract from the purpose of illustrating principles.

The selected references listed at the end of this book were helpful to the authors as they wrote and may serve the reader in the same way.

The Problem

Consider the following operating room scene:

"Knife"

The scrub nurse snaps the knife handle into the surgeon's outstretched right palm. The surgeon places the blade on the abdominal skin below the costal margin near the midline. He looks over the drapes to the anesthesiologist. "OK to start?"

The surgeon begins his incision but stops midway down the right costal margin. His first assistant has not applied skin traction below the incision equal to his own traction above. The incision is beveled and skewing toward the costal edge. He adjusts the assistant and continues the incision, leaving a small "V" at the junction of the two cuts.

The first assistant, a junior resident eager to do something and impress the surgeon, requests hemostats and attacks active bleeders. He desperately clamps a wad of tissue as an arterial pumper disappears in the accumulating pool of blood. The surgeon, meanwhile, takes a pad and covers the field. He grasps the assistant's wrist and firmly places his hand over the pad, immobilizing him. He gradually unfolds the pad and shows the resident how to secure bleeders one at a time.

"Deep knife, blunt rakes"

The surgeon places the rakes in the abundant subcutaneous fat for his assistant to hold.

The resident, upset about his awkward performance on the subcutaneous bleeders, is distracted and does not pull evenly with both rakes. As a result, the incisions down through fat become a series of jagged steps as the surgeon tries to compensate for the shifting position of his target.

"Why do I always get stuck with the junior residents?" mutters the surgeon.

The resident's embarrassment is mixed with anger.

The patient was concerned about the scar so the surgeon has made the smallest incision he thinks he can work through.

The abdomen is opened and body wall retractors are placed for the assistant and medical student to hold. The surgeon does a cursory local exploration and begins freeing omental adhesions at the fundus of the gallbladder. Progress is slow. The surgeon pushes the second assistant to his left to get elbow room because he is working in a hole. The displaced assistant loses his grip on the body wall retractor and it slips out. The surgeon roughly replaces the retractor on the unprotected abdominal wall and commands the assistant to pull harder.

"Large clamp, narrow Deaver"

Gradually the gallbladder is exposed and the fundus is clamped for traction. The narrow Deaver is placed on the underside of the liver to the left of the gallbladder. Deep lap pads are placed and retracted.

"Long Metz"

The surgeon begins to dissect the edge of the hepatoduodenal ligament and looks for the cystic duct.

"Give me traction"

The first assistant has his left hand on the pad over the duodenum. In order to understand what he is to retract, he leans over the obese patient to peer into the deep hole where the surgeon is working. In the process his head clunks solidly into the surgeon's over the hole. The surgeon, frustrated by the difficulties, explodes at the hapless resident.

The surgeon finally isolates the cystic duct. The position of the cystic artery is unclear. As the surgeon dissects, the points of his right-angle clamps tear a vessel and blood wells up in the hole.

"Toe in your retractor," he yells at the medical student. His arms cramped from the lengthy dissection, the student tips the retractor up and leans back. The tip of the retractor tears a small rent in the liver, which begins to bleed profusely.

The surgeon breaks into a cold sweat, shouts at the nurse for a long clamp. The nurse, flustered by the tension in the room, hands him a long right angle instead of the tonsil clamp he expected. A heated exchange follows.

The anesthesiologist looks up, concerned by the surgeon's panic. He asks for an assessment of the situation as the surgeon blindly clamps for the bleeding vessel in the dark well of blood.

The surgeon quickly packs lap pads into the wound and realizes that he has to extend his incision to gain adequate exposure.

When the bleeding is finally controlled, the surgeon discovers that he has clamped part of the common duct.

That such a scenario ever occurs is unfortunate. These and other errors can turn a straightforward case into a nightmare followed by a tragedy. Isolated breaks in technique must be expected as part of the learning process. Errors, however, have a way of compounding themselves, and the cascade effect leads to disaster. Adherence to the following principles minimizes the occurrence of such errors.

The Principles

I. First do no harm!
II. The surgeon's quality
   A. Behavior pattern
      1. Pay compulsive attention to detail
      2. Make logical decisions
      3. Exercise self-control
      4. Act consistently under stress
      5. Show maturity
      6. Demonstrate leadership
   B. Manual proficiency
      1. Natural dexterity
      2. Practiced skills
      3. Economy of motion
   C. Preparation
      1. Didactic knowledge including anatomy and pathophysiology
      2. Know surgical procedures
      3. Study the patient: operate at the proper time; not too early or too late
      4. Prepare the patient psychologically and physically

5. Arrange for surgery
   a) Appropriate assistants
   b) Special instruments
   c) Special studies (e. g., X-ray films)
   d) Consultant support
   e) Post-op facilities (e. g., ICU)
D. Post-op care: The operation is a brief event in the total care of a patient

III. Asepsis
   A. Follow sterile technique rigorously
   B. Avoid environment favorable to bacteria
      1. Do not leave culture media in the wound
         a) Minimize dead tissue
            i) No mass ligature
            ii) Minimal cautery
            iii) Preserve blood supply
            iv) Irrigate to debride mechanically
         b) Minimize blood accumulation by careful hemostasis
         c) Dissect carefully to minimize raw surfaces that ooze serum
         d) Place drains when fluid is likely to collect
      2. Eliminate dead space where culture media accumulate
      3. Minimize foreign material left in the wound
      4. Leave high-risk wounds open to granulate initially
   C. Decrease the inoculum of bacteria present during surgery
      1. Sterilize sources of contamination such as bowel
      2. Work efficiently to decrease exposure time and probability of contamination
      3. Use antibiotics appropriately
         a) Prophylactically when there is a high risk of infection or when the consequences of infection could be disastrous
         b) Therapeutically for existing contamination
      4. Dilute bacteria to extinction by copious irrigation
      5. Minimize movement and talking in the operating room
   D. Ensure that host resistance is at normal levels; correct pre-op metabolic, nutritional, and drug-induced problems

IV. Tissue handling
   A. Manipulations
      1. Gentle

2. Clean, decisive movements
3. Approximate tissue, do not strangulate it with sutures
4. Use proper instruments
5. No mass ligature
   B. Dissection
      1. Sharp
      2. Follow anatomic planes
      3. Preserve functional tissue and keep blood supply intact
      4. Mobilize only what can be seen
   C. Protect tissue
      1. Keep it moist
      2. Minimize exposure time
      3. Minimize electrocoagulation

V. Hemostasis
   A. Screen preoperatively for coagulation defects
   B. Ensure secure ties
      1. Square knots
      2. The proper number of knots for the material
      3. Suture or double ligation of high-risk vessels
   C. Coagulate precisely to prevent damage to surrounding tissues
   D. Use appropriate clamps to hold vessels securely without injuring adjacent tissue
      1. Grasp the minimal tissue necessary
      2. Choose the correct size clamp for the job
   E. Secure proximal control of major vessels first

VI. Exposure
   A. Positions
      1. Patient
      2. Surgeon
      3. Assistants
   B. Focus and readjust light as the operative field changes
   C. Incision
      1. Make it large enough to allow visibility and maneuverability
      2. Take into account anatomic obstacles when placing it
   D. Retraction is a key to exposure; an adequate incision allows gentle retraction that does not damage tissue
   E. The length of instruments must reflect the depth of the structure on which they are used; they should also keep hands out of the line of vision

First Do No Harm

The historical admonition to the physician to "first do no harm" is implemented through application of the other principles. References to preventive and precautionary maneuvers occur throughout the book. ⟡ ⁀

The Surgeon

At first glance it may seem unorthodox to include attributes of the surgeon with principles of technique. As the story unfolds, however, it will become clear how the surgeon's character is part of his technique. Some attributes of the good surgeon are behavior patterns and personality traits. Attention to details, calm logical thought under stress, and effective leadership constitute surgical maturity. One example of maturity is the ability to accept advice from a more experienced surgeon without feeling threatened.

Manual proficiency can be developed and refined, but it helps if the student contemplating a surgical career is naturally dexterous. Speed is not an end in itself and may lead to errors. It is lack of wasted moves that allows rapid completion of a case, not fast movement. Every good surgeon establishes a rhythm and tries to maintain his ideal pace. Technically impeccable, gentle surgery makes a huge contribution to the outcome of an operation and to the patient's recovery.

The adage that genius is 99% perspiration and 1% inspiration holds true for surgery. Preparation for an operation includes didactic knowledge and careful study of the patient; open communication with the patient is vital at every stage to win and hold the patient's trust. Arrangements must be made for assistance, special equipment, and specialty support. The work of treating a surgical patient begins long before the operation and continues long after.

Asepsis

Asepsis involves more than meticulous sterile technique. The conditions favorable to bacterial growth must be avoided. Dead tissue, collection of blood or serum, and the presence of foreign material all foster bacterial growth. Rough manipulation, poor hemostasis, and the presence of "dead" space promote hematoma and seroma formation. Minimizing the inoculum of bacteria involves efficient surgery, prophylactic cleansing of contaminated areas, and the appropriate use of antibiotics. Endogenous sour-

ces of contamination (bowel content, infected bile, abscess) are more significant and more difficult to control than exogenous sources. Host resistance is affected by nutrition and may be improved by appropriate preoperative alimentation. The interdependence of these principles of technique is evidenced throughout the book.

Tissue Handling

The principles listed under this heading have one common goal: to kill as few cells as possible. This aspect of surgical technique is emphasized in virtually every chapter of the book.

Hemostasis

Inadequate hemostasis may result in minor ecchymosis following a breast biopsy or exsanguinating hemorrhage after splenectomy. Preoperative evaluation of clotting parameters is a vital precaution. A set of principles pertaining to knots serves as a guide to tying accurate, secure square knots. Additional comments on knot tying are found in the chapter on surgical maneuvers.

The use of clamps and cautery is also discussed. Proximal control of major vessels is a basic principle of vascular surgery.

Exposure

The last group of principles in the outline deals with the elements of exposure. Illumination, physical access, and an unobstructed view must be kept optimal through constant readjustment.

Because of poor tissue reflectance and contrast, operating-room lights must deliver intense illumination just below the level of significant radiant energy heat transfer to tissue. Most American operating-room lights focus at about 42 inches, with a variable diameter field that is most intense at its center. A 10- to 12-inch depth of focus allows even illumination in a deep wound. Outside of this local area, the light appears as a ring with a dark center.

Eyestrain can occur because of glare (shiny instruments, white sponges, drapes) and disproportionally low surrounding light. Environmental light should ideally be one third the level of the task lighting.

To minimize shadows, light sources are made diffuse by using multiple lights or a large reflector. Directing lights around personnel and overlapping the fields also help, as do fiberoptic headlights.

Although individual lights meet heat transfer specifications, the effect of multiple lights is additive (as you can feel by holding your hand at such a focal point). Frequent irrigation is a necessary precaution.

Lights may need to be adjusted as the focus of attention in the operative field changes. The fixture's gimbals should be snug enough to hold the light's position without drifting.

Principles of exposure are laid out in the chapters on instruments, manipulations, and the surgical assistant and are demonstrated with each procedure in Part II.

The principles cannot be ranked by priority. They are equally important and interdependent. A unified concept of good surgical technique should emerge from learning the fundamentals.

Chapter 1

Historical Notes on Surgical Technique

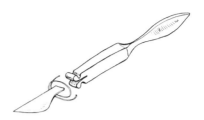

The story of surgery from prehistoric times up to the modern era is in large measure the story of traumatic wounds. Of the earliest surgery we know little, but we might guess that it consisted of caring for traumatic wounds and the extraction of projectile points. Wounds were probably treated with a poultice and allowed to heal by secondary intention. Hemostasis was unknown, and hemorrhage often meant death.

The battlefield, with its renowned capacity for creating traumatic wounds in great numbers, has always figured prominently in the advance of surgical technique. It has been stated in many ways that young surgeons are the only ones who gain from warfare because they have an opportunity to develop their surgical skills much more rapidly than they might in the civilian practice of surgery. The modern hospital derives from the first military hospitals, established by the Romans for their soldiers in distant northern campaigns. The battlefield was also the stage for some of Paré's epochal advances at the dawn of the modern era.

We have fragmentary but often fascinating evidence of the ingenuity of ancient surgeons. In a review of the surgical techniques employed in ancient times (such as the one by Majno), one finds surprising similarities to the practices of today, even though there is great contrast between ancient and recent understanding of the pathophysiology of disease and injury.

The Prehistoric Period

Although archeologists and historians may argue over whether castration of bulls or trepanation of the human skull was the first surgical procedure, the latter is more pertinent to this review. An operation to remove a portion of the skull may have been performed as far back as 10,000 B.C. This bold act, which is still done today, was performed by many primitive peoples, including extensive practice by the Incas of Peru. In many instances the opening in an ancient skull is associated with a fracture line and was done to relieve the effect of trauma. In such cases we can imagine the assistant grasping the hair on either side to retract the scalp (Fig. 1.1) as the surgeon cuts with a razor-sharp flaked flint tool. (A noted anthropologist once demonstrated his belief in the superiority of the fracture-flaked edge over surgical steel by insisting that his surgeon perform his appendectomy using a tool he had so fashioned.) When trepanation was done for magical reasons rather than trauma, we can assume that additional assistants were required to hold down the conscious patient.

One method of creating the opening was cutting a circular groove. The procedure was also done by scraping, by cutting intersecting lines, and by drilling a circle of small holes. When the Greeks employed this last method, they observed the precaution of

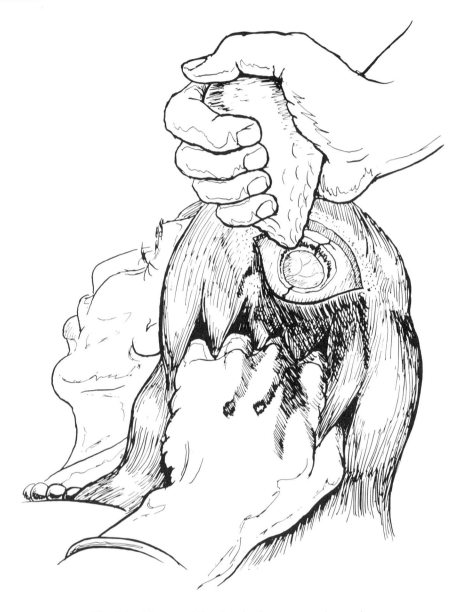

Fig. 1.1   After completing the circular groove and removing a
disc of bone, the surgeon smooths the edges of the opening.

drilling slowly since such drills were also used for
starting fires and generated considerable heat. Evidence of healing in many cases attests to the success
of trepanation.

The surgical art of trepanning did not change
appreciably for thousands of years and was still practiced at the turn of this century among more primitive
peoples. Ironically, in civilized countries iatrogenic
infection made mortality from this procedure pro-
hibitive through the 19th century.

Mesopotamia

Approximately 5000 years ago in southern Mesopotamia (now Iraq), the Sumerians developed writing. In the clay tablets constituting the earliest written history, there are only rare references to the surgery of the day. We know that castration of animals and humans was performed. We can also deduce that surgery was extremely risky to both the patient and the surgeon. Hammurabi's Code of ca. 1700 B.C. specifies that the fee for a lifesaving operation done with a bronze lancet shall be ten shekels of silver. If the same operation results in the death of the patient, "they shall cut off [the physician's] hand."

One remarkable tablet clearly describes fluctuation and the treatment of a scalp abscess. It indicates that if the swelling does not yield when pressed with the finger, heat should be applied until it does. Then it may be incised and drained.

Egypt

The first hieroglyphs appeared around 2900 B.C., 200 years after the earliest Sumerian tablets. We have no evidence that the medicine practiced by one culture was influenced by the other. The earliest recorded Egyptian surgical procedure is circumcision, depicted on a bas-relief ca. 2250 B.C.; it was probably done with a stone blade. The largest concentration of papyri concerning medicine appears in the Middle Kingdom (1900–1200 B.C.), and from these we know that Egyptian physicians specialized in various areas of the body. Surgery was concerned mainly with the treatment of wounds. The Ebers papyrus mentions four types of surgical blade. One was flint and another of reed, and although the other two cannot be deciphered, we can assume that one was of metal (bronze) because the Smith papyrus describes using a red-hot knife to cut and cauterize vessels simultaneously. This is the first recorded use of cautery for hemostasis.

The Egyptians used both sutures and tapes (Fig. 1.2) to close wounds, and differentiated between healthy and unhealthy wounds. The Smith papyrus contains an instruction to use sutures first. If on the first day the wound falls apart, reapproximate with tapes; if that fails, leave the wound open.

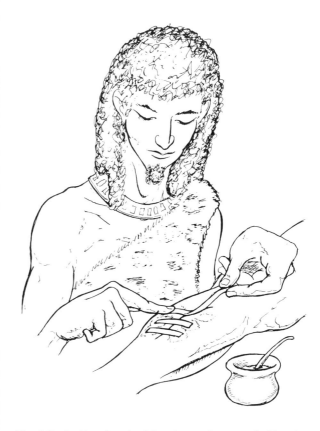

Fig. 1.2 An Egyptian physician closes a leg wound with strips of linen and acacia gum adhesive.

Greece

Asklepios was a chief of Thessaly who fought in the Trojan war and, with his sons, helped treat the Greeks' battle wounds. The legend of his medical powers grew in succeeding centuries and led to the establishment of a religious cult ca. 700 B.C. Seeking a miraculous cure, the sick flocked to the temples of Asklepios, and from this cult a secular branch arose to deal with the actual treatment of patients. From the school of medicine on the island of Cos, Hippocrates (460–380 B.C.) emerged. Hippocrates applied Greek rationality and high ideals to medicine and surgery. He anticipated Semmelweis by over 2000 years in insisting that his followers keep their hands and nails meticulously clean. They filtered or boiled water before using it to wash wounds and used only fresh linen for dressings. They even wrote about operating theater lighting, the patient's position, the surgeon's position, and instrument care. Surgery took a giant, temporary step forward; had the subsequent history of Europe been less calamitous, the foundations might have been laid for modern practice.

The Hippocratic procedure for draining an empyema (Figs. 1.3–1.7) could be a description of the modern procedure. Trepanation for skull fracture was performed by the Greeks, as were a variety of minor procedures. Cautery was the only method of hemostasis until a short time after Hippocrates.

Like the Mesopotamians, the Hippocratic physicians left us instructions for treatment of an abscess. The Greeks coated an abscess with a thin layer of wet potter's clay. The clay dried first at the hottest point (which should correspond with the most tender point), and the skin was then washed and incised.

Many of the Hippocratic texts have been lost, but we know of them indirectly through their influence on medicine in Alexandria and Rome.

Before continuing with the progress of Western medicine, let us briefly turn East.

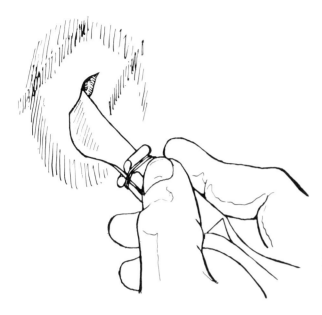

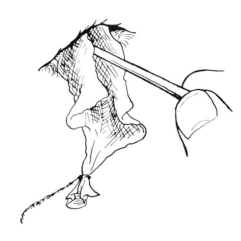

Fig. 1.5   A piece of linen tagged with thread is pushed into the opening with a probe. The linen is removed daily to allow drainage.

Fig. 1.3   The physician incises the skin between the ribs at the hottest point, using a round-bladed knife. The cut is made as low as possible to let the pus flow out freely.

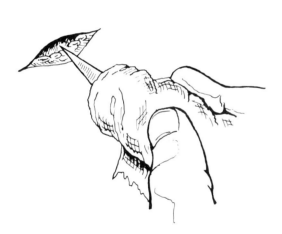

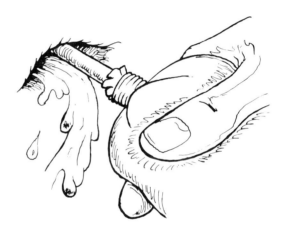

Fig. 1.6   On the tenth day, when the drainage has diminished, warm wine and oil are injected and left for 12 hours.

Fig. 1.4   With a pointed blade wrapped in cloth to within a thumbnail's distance of the point, the physician punctures the chest cavity.

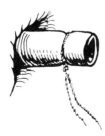

Fig. 1.7   A hollow tin drain is inserted and is cut shorter as the wound heals.

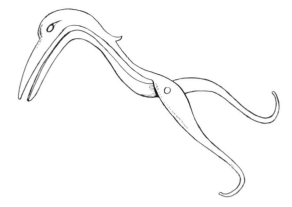

Fig. 1.8   The heron-mouth forceps could extract a deep-seated foreign body.

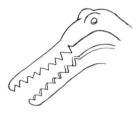

Fig. 1.9   This toothed forceps is in the form of a crocodile head.

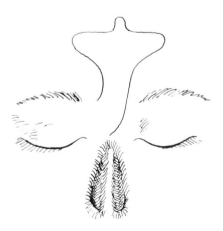

Fig. 1.10   A skin flap is mobilized from the forehead.

India

Although sutures were used in China from the second century B.C., Chinese surgery had very low status and made little progress. In contrast, surgery flourished in India, particularly plastic and reconstructive surgery of the face. The major surgical teachings originated with Sushruta and were transmitted in the form of memorized doctrine. The grasping ends of surgical tools, made in the form of animal heads (Fig. 1.8 and 1.9), were designed for specific purposes such as extracting arrow heads, again demonstrating the progress of surgery as an effect of warfare. In a remarkable parallel to Hippocrates' trick using potter's clay, the legendary physician Sushruta recommended clarified butter and earth be applied over the suspected location of an embedded arrowhead. Where the mixture dried first would be the hottest point, overlying the arrowhead and presumably an abscess.

Amputation of ears and noses, both as a result of warfare and also as punitive measures, led Sushruta to devise pedicle flaps for reconstruction (Figs. 1.10 and 1.11). The rich blood supply and low risk of infection of the face undoubtedly contributed to the success of these procedures.

Sushruta outlined a series of exercises for the technical training of novice surgeons. These included incising a vegetable (Fig. 1.12), lancing a leather bag full of muck to simulate an abscess (Fig. 1.13), picking seeds out of a fruit with surgical forceps (Fig. 1.14), probing in rotten wood (Fig. 1.15), suturing on cloth (Fig. 1.16), and cauterizing raw meat (Fig. 1.17).

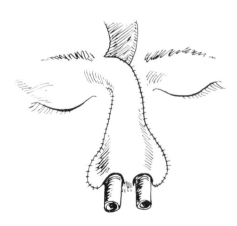

Fig. 1.11   The flap is rotated and sutured into the nasal defect after the edges of the defect are freshly incised.

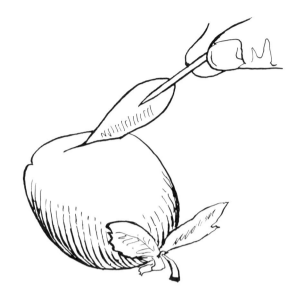

Fig. 1.12

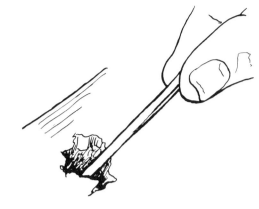

Fig. 1.15

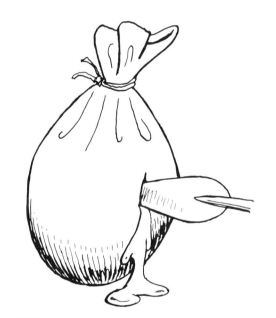

Fig. 1.13

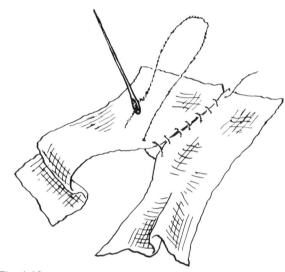

Fig. 1.16

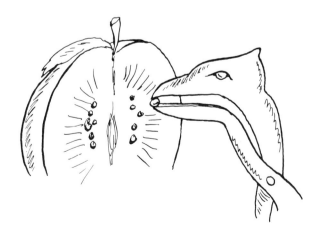

Fig. 1.14

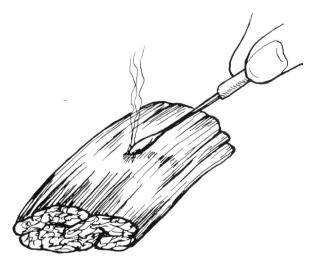

Fig. 1.17

Alexandria

The city Alexander founded in Egypt grew while Rome was consolidating its empire, and Greek medicine flourished in its university. Scientific dissection of animals and humans led to the performance of major surgery (excision of goiter, even laparotomy) in the last centuries B.C. A major innovation attributed to the Alexandrian school was the use of ligatures to tie individual blood vessels (although the concepts of circulation and exsanguination were still not known).

Rome

Greek medicine arrived in Rome by the direct infusion of Greek physicians and via Alexandria. Early in the first century A.D., Celsus, a chronicler, not a physician, recorded the firm establishment of Greek surgery in Rome. Both Hippocratic ideas and Greek instruments were adopted wholesale. A rich collection of Roman surgical instruments survives, including a large number buried at Pompeii when Vesuvius erupted ca. 79 A.D. Among these are scalpel handles with blunt dissecting ends (Fig. 1.18), forceps (Fig. 1.19), and probes (Fig. 1.20). It is interesting to note the variety of hemostatic clamps that had evolved since the Alexandrians described ligating individual vessels (Figs. 1.21 and 1.22). Hook retractors (Fig. 1.23) suggest an increasing technical sophistication in Roman surgery.

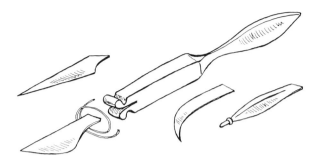

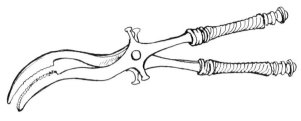

Fig. 1.21   The crosspieces of this clamp could have been tied together to keep the jaws locked.

Fig. 1.18   Blades were probably fastened to the scalpel handle using wire or thread. Pointed, bellied, falciform (sickle-shaped), and probe-tipped fistula blades are shown.

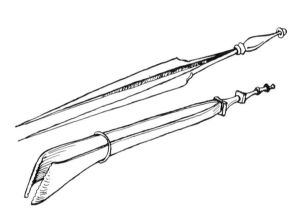

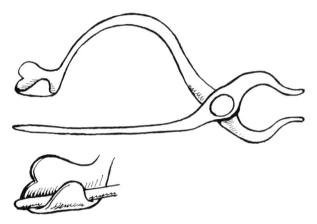

Fig. 1.19   The forceps with the sliding ring, found at Pompeii, may have served as a hemostat.

Fig. 1.22   This Gallo-Roman clamp (first to third century a.d.) has a locking handle.

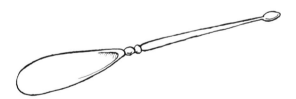

Fig. 1.20   The Greeks and Romans made wide use of probes.

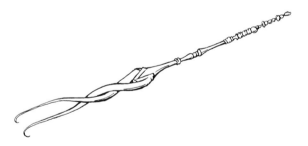

Fig. 1.23   This fine set of hooks is one of the earliest retractors known.

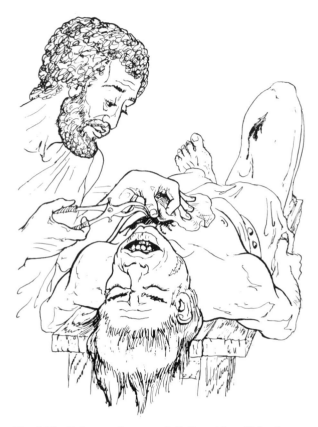

Fig. 1.24   Galen may have used silk thread from China for ligatures.

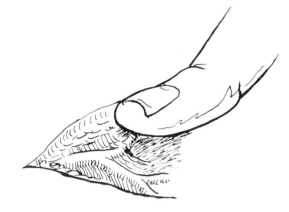

Fig. 1.25   The simplest of Galen's hemostatic manuevers was direct pressure.

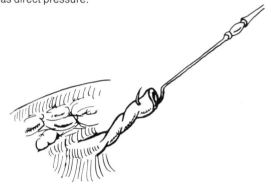

Fig. 1.26   This maneuver of Galen's is described again by Halsted in 1913.

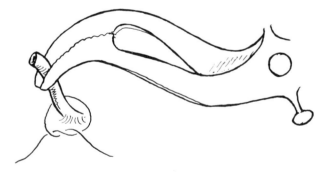

Fig. 1.27   Grasping and tying involved more complex skills.

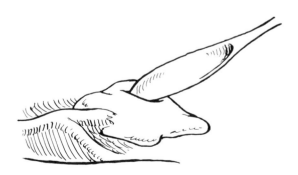

Fig. 1.28   Application of styptics may have been a holdover from more ancient practices.

Galen (130–200 A.D.) studied Greek medicine in Pergamon and Alexandria. He acted as surgeon to wounded gladiators in Pergamon (Fig. 1.24) and later became court physician to Marcus Aurelius in Rome. His voluminous writings became the mainstay of Western medicine for 1500 years. He recognized that fascia should be included in sutures reapproximating muscle, he sutured tendons, and (following the Hippocratic teaching) he recognized that pus was not necessary for healing. His surgical technique included keeping exposed tissue moist, debriding macerated tissue before suturing, and controlling bleeding vessels. Galen describes four methods of hemostasis: direct pressure on the bleeding vessel (Fig. 1.25), twisting the vessel with a hook (Fig. 1.26), grasping the vessel with forceps and tying (Fig. 1.27), and applying styptics (Fig. 1.28). He employed assistants to compress multiple bleeding points and elevated the bleeding part. The compression, he said, should be done gently, without causing pain.

Surgery made little progress during the Dark Ages. Even so basic a technique as hemostasis received no attention. In his autobiography, Benvenuto Cellini writes of his brother's death in 1529: The "arquebusier . . . fired . . . and hit [my brother] above the knee of his right leg." The "wound had been dressed," but he "lost blood so copiously, for nothing could be done to stop it," that he died the following morning.

Beyond the Classical Period

From the decline of Rome to the end of the 19th century, surgery made tentative rather than dramatic advances. To put in perspective the development of surgical technique during this period, one may look to a series of remarkable individuals who assessed objectively what they saw and had the courage to contradict erroneous notions embedded in tradition. The most significant advances were in the areas of anatomy and military surgery. Since trauma presented the most urgent demand for surgical remedies, the battlefield served as the classroom for most of these innovators. Persistent controversies waxed and waned over these years: the role of pus in wound healing, cautery vs. the knife, the use of ligature vs. cautery for hemostasis. The anatomists, especially at the time of the Renaissance, made major contributions to the scientific basis of surgery. This period must be viewed as a lag phase compared to the revolutionary changes precipitated by the advent of asepsis and anesthesia in the 19th century. Let us look briefly at some of the actors who left their mark on surgery prior to the 20th century.

Arabic Physicians

The Persian physician Rhazes (Fig. 1.29), born in 852 A.D., wrote extensively and was one of those who preserved the Greek medical legacy by translating it into Arabic. One of his own numerous contributions to surgery grew out of his experience as a lute player. Drawing on his knowledge of animal gut lute strings, he used that material as a suture to repair abdominal wounds. His countryman Avicenna (b. 980 A.D.) was also a renowned physician and prolific writer. In surgery Avicenna felt that cautery was always preferable to the knife. His influence on surgery, however, was not all positive. He did surgery a disservice by considering it a separate, inferior branch of medi-

cine. Albucasis (b. 936 A.D.), a Spaniard, also wrote extensively in Arabic on his medical and surgical experience. Included in his works are some of the earliest illustrations of surgical and dental instruments. Unlike Avicenna, he championed the use of cutting instruments as well as cautery in surgery.

No new anatomical insights derive from this period because Islam forbade dissection. As the cultural domination of Islam was declining, medical schools were being established throughout Europe and the succeeding generations of surgeons sought the formal education offered there.

The Academics

Medical schools appeared in Paris, Montpellier, Salerno, Bologna, Padua, Milan, and Britain between the 11th and 13th centuries. Prominent among the academic writings of this period was a body of surgical literature that evolved in Italy, incorporating the teachings of Roger Frugardi of Palermo and his pupil, Roland of Parma. In dealing with the ubiquitous traumatic wound, they recommended (again) the use of ligatures for bleeding vessels that could not be stopped by cautery or styptics. The warfare of the day often had the head as a prime target. From treating these injuries they formulated recommendations for diagnosing skull fractures by finger palpa-

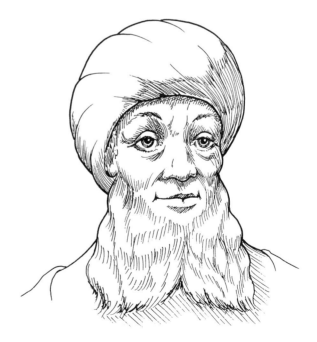

Fig. 1.29   The Persian physician Rhazes helped preserve the legacy of Greek medicine by translating Greek works into Arabic and made significant contributions of his own.

tion, debriding loose bone fragments, and controlling scalp bleeding. Although the surgeons of the time became skilled at one commonly performed major operation, amputation, the limits of surgery remained remarkably unchanged from Egyptian practice thousands of years before, as evidenced by the statement, "If a man is wounded in the heart, lung, liver, or diaphragm, we do not undertake his treatment." These writings passed on the premise that suppuration, "laudable pus," was necessary for wounds to heal.

The academically trained friar-surgeon Theodoric published a treatise in 1266 in which he firmly stated that pus was not only unnecessary for wound healing but was destructive. This set up the controversy that was to simmer over the next five centuries. Theodoric was supported by some like Henri de Mondeville, lecturer in anatomy in Montpellier, who advocated the clean treatment of wounds. He was condemned by others such as Guy de Chauliac, whose opinions, unfortunately, prevailed.

Like many medical students of his day, Guy de Chauliac traveled from university to university for instruction. His time at Paris, Montpellier, Toulouse, and Bologna made him one of the best educated surgeons of his era. de Chauliac achieved a preeminent position in surgery, and his text, *La Grande Chirurgie,* published in 1363, influenced the practice of surgery for the next 200 years. While giving due respect to venerable surgical teachings, he considered that body of knowledge subject to revision and a starting point for adding new information. He excelled in the treatment of traumatic wounds and fractures and recommended the open treatment of dirty wounds. de Chauliac also recognized the importance of anatomy to the surgeon. He compared a surgeon ignorant of anatomy to a blind man trying to cut a log. More than 100 years later, the study of anatomy finally flourished at the time of the Renaissance.

The Anatomists

The fertile environment of the Renaissance nurtured many new ideas. The artists of the period embraced the philosophy that art should be a faithful representation of nature, and artist-anatomists such as Leonardo da Vinci acquired their knowledge through human cadaver dissection. Their unpublished work had no direct influence on medicine, but the precedents they established set the stage for the work of Andreas Vesalius.

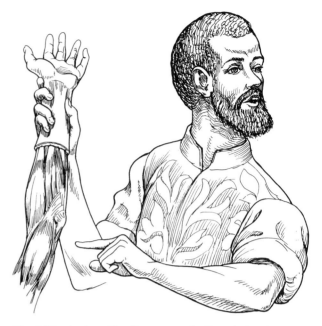

Fig. 1.30   Andreas Vesalius personally dissected and demonstrated anatomy. He published and disseminated monumental works that are both accurate and beautiful.

Vesalius was born in Brussels in 1514, five years before the death of Leonardo. He demonstrated his skill as a dissector at the University of Paris and subsequently received his medical degree from the University of Padua, a center of the blossoming scientific renaissance. He broke with tradition and descended from the lecturer's platform to personally perform dissections and demonstrate anatomy (Fig. 1.30). He gained great popularity and often illustrated his lectures with large drawings that he drew himself. Encouraged by the response to these illustrations, he sought out his countryman, Jan Stefan van Kalkar, an art student at Titian's workshop in nearby Venice. Combining his own illustrations with van Kalkar's in his first publication, *Tabulae Anatomicae Sex* (1538), he set a new standard in anatomical illustration. His subsequent works are landmarks of anatomy and art. At last the human body had been carefully explored and Galen's animal-derived misconceptions had been corrected. Equally important, the information was disseminated in printed form in the classic *De Fabrica Humani Corporis* of 1543.

Paré and the 16th Century

Ambroise Paré (b. 1509) started his medical career as a barber-surgeon's apprentice and then worked as a house surgeon in Paris' largest hospital, the Hôtel Dieu, to expand his surgical knowledge. At age 26 Paré became a military surgeon and traveled with the

French armies. Gunshot wounds were becoming a prevalent injury, and the wounds were thought to be poisoned by gunpowder. To counteract the poison, the wounds were cauterized with boiling oil. During the French retreat from Turin in 1536, the number of casualties exceeded the available supply of oil. With great trepidation Paré treated the remaining wounds with a paste of egg yolks and oil of roses in turpentine (Fig. 1.31). To his amazement the noncauterized wounds fared much better. He recognized the importance of his observation and convinced his contemporaries of its validity. He went on to become surgeon-in-chief to four French kings. He wrote extensively and translated Vesalius' works into French. His many contributions to surgery include the introduction of the ligature for bleeding vessels during amputation and his emphasis on rational simplicity and cleanliness.

One must keep in mind that outstanding surgeons like Paré did not exist in a vacuum and that numerous contemporaries also made significant contributions. William Clowes of Elizabethan England achieved good results with common sense and minimal use of cautery. He successfully treated the evisceration of a naval gunner in 1540 by amputating the omentum, replacing the gut, and suturing the abdominal

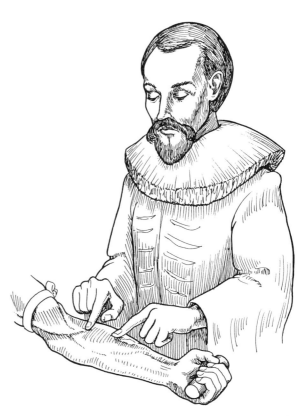

Fig. 1.32   William Harvey sought rigorous scientific proofs in living organisms and was the founder of experimental physiology.

wound. Alexander Read, another Briton, was a quick and skillful surgeon who devised innovative suturing techniques and was one of the earliest experimental surgeons. He removed the spleen of a dog, and the dog survived, laying to rest the controversy over whether or not the spleen was necessary for life. Johann Scultetus of Ulm was another great illustrator of surgery, who published extensive works on instrumentation and surgical procedures. The combined contributions of these few well-known and many lesser-known surgeons led to the increasing role of science in surgery.

Surgical Scientists

William Harvey received his bachelor's degree from Cambridge College and in 1597 at age 19 went to Padua to study anatomy under Fabricius, who in turn was taught by Fallopius, Vesalius' chief pupil. Fabricius was studying the venous valves at the time and postulated that their purpose was to prevent accumulation of blood in the extremities during the Galenic tidal ebb and flow. The work of Fabricius and others served as a starting point for Harvey's investigations over the ensuing years (Fig. 1.33).

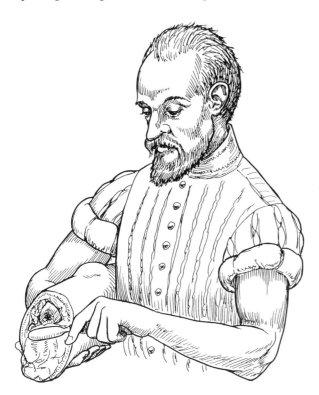

Fig. 1.31   Ambroise Paré stressed simplicity and cleanliness in surgical treatment and overturned the practice of cauterizing wounds with boiling oil.

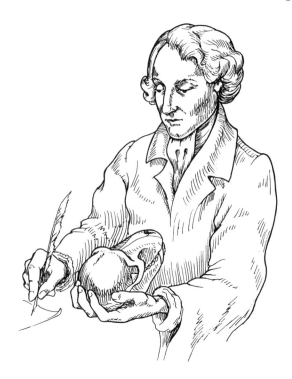

Fig. 1.33   John Hunter introduced scientific method into surgery and applied to clinical practice those insights gained from his observations of nature.

Harvey made precise quantitative measurements in live animal experiments and reintroduced vivisection to the science of his time. (A millenium earlier Galen had silenced the squeals of a pig by cutting the recurrent laryngeal nerve). Harvey observed the sequential contraction of atria and ventricles, particularly noticeable in slower beating lower vertebrate hearts; he watched the heart empty and turn pale when its venous supply was compressed and watched it dilate when its outflow was obstructed. By an exhaustive and varied set of experimental proofs, he demonstrated that the volume of blood exiting the heart was far in excess of what could be supplied by food and that blood must flow in a circle. He published his findings in 1628. His original experiments and clear logic set a standard for what would eventually become experimental physiology. Men such as John Hunter would later apply this methodology to surgery.

John Hunter, the youngest of ten children, came to London in 1748 to begin his surgical studies. He was aided by his respected obstetrician-anatomist brother William. John had an insatiable curiosity about living things, and he dissected and collected specimens of innumerable species over his lifetime (Fig. 1.33). From his studies he established general principles that could then be applied to interpret individual cases. He brought this approach to surgery in a revolutionary reversal of traditional methods. Rather than describing an isolated disease and its particular surgical remedy, he insisted that his students understand the principles of the pathology, and then the nature of the condition and its treatment would naturally follow.

In 1785 he put his observations and principles to work in a dramatic surgical demonstration. He had observed that when deer shed and regrew antlers, the central artery withered and its function was assumed by numerous collaterals. He correctly reasoned that the collateral vessels around the knee would maintain the viability of the lower leg if the flow to an aneurysmal popliteal artery were interrupted. He had also experimentally established that it was pulsations that caused the continual dilatation of the aneurysm and that the clot forming the mass of the sac would be resorbed if the flow of fresh blood was cut off. He ligated the femoral artery above the knee (in the canal that now bears his name) and proved his hypothesis correct. As Harvey founded experimental physiology, Hunter established experimental and surgical pathology as a science.

At the same time that surgical science advanced, the necessities of warfare found surgeons to meet the age-old challenge of man's self-inflicted trauma. One of the most outstanding of these men was Dominique Jean Larrey, a surgeon of Napoleon's army, who stressed the delivery of aid to the wounded in the midst of battle and instituted mobile hospitals and "flying ambulances." He was a proponent of immediate amputation after injury.

Superimposed on the achievements of all these men, the advent of anesthesia and aseptic practice during the 19th century set the stage for an explosive growth of surgery.

Anesthesia and Asepsis

Ether was introduced by the dentist William Morton of Boston, who gave the first public demonstration in 1846. James Young Simpson, Professor of Midwifery at Edinburgh, introduced chloroform the next year and general anesthesia became accepted practice over the next decade. With speed no longer essential to minimize pain, men such as Theodor Kocher and William Halsted were able to dramatically extend the range of surgical operations and emphasize careful, methodical technique and gentle tissue handling. The results might still have been compromised by infection if other perceptive individuals had not made their own discoveries at the same time.

Alexander Gordon of Aberdeen and Ignaz Semmelweis of Vienna observed that puerperal sepsis seemed to be spread from patient to patient by the attending physician. Karl Haller, a surgeon who practiced at the Allgemeines Krankenhaus with Semmelweis, extrapolated the cause-and-effect relationship of unsanitary practices to surgical infections in 1849. These early intimations of infectious disease had little impact on surgical practice. In 1865 Pasteur demonstrated that fermentation and putrefaction were caused by microorganisms in the air. This clue led Joseph Lister in 1867 to use carbolic acid in the first attempts at surgical antisepsis. Von Bergmann in Germany led the way in transforming antisepsis to an aseptic technique.

Anesthesia, asepsis, antibiotics, and whole blood transfusion have allowed the surgeon to refine and perfect surgical technique. The technique combined with the other factors produces safe surgery and routinely good results. That surgical technique is the focus of this book.

Chapter 2

Wound Healing and Surgical Technique

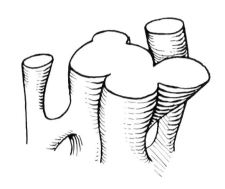

A major determinant of a patient's recovery is the healing of the wounds created during an operation. In order to understand the impact of surgical technique on healing, it is helpful to review the fundamentals of wound repair. The first part of this chapter is a brief overview of the histochemical aspects of repair and the practical implications of this process. Surgical technique, wound management, and skin grafting are discussed in the second part of this chapter.

Histochemical Aspects of Repair

Vascular Response to Injury

Immediately after injury there is vasoconstriction in the local microcirculation. Platelets bind to exposed collagen and interact with thrombin to initiate clotting. The resulting clot acts as a tissue adhesive and provides a fibrin framework for later events. The clot, however, provides poor protection for the underlying tissue.

After about 10 minutes, active vasodilation occurs, caused by several factors. Histamine, primarily from mast cells, has a short-acting (30 minutes) effect on small-vessel permeability. The venules (20–30 μ) rather than capillaries (4–7 μ) are the primary vessels affected. Endothelial cells separate, perhaps by rounding under the influence of histamine and other vasoactive substances. Basement membrane is exposed and plasma begins to leak. Later in the inflammatory response, when granulocytes have extravasated, the kallikrein system and prostaglandins exert a continuing effect on microvascular dilation and permeability. The release of proteolytic enzymes futher compromises microvascular integrity.

Lymphatics are more fragile than blood vessels. Fibrin plugs lymphatics and blocks drainage from the area of the injury, localizing the inflammatory process. Later, activation of fibrinolytic enzymes clears the blocked lymphatic channels (see Fig. 2.1).

Cellular Response

Within hours of injury white cells begin to adhere to microvascular endothelium and migrate into the area of injury. Various factors attract cells into the wound, including C5a (the fifth component of complement), prostaglandin E_1 and E_2, and fibrin.

Polymorphonuclear leukocytes (polys) predominate in the first 2–3 days. They phagocytize debris and bacteria. The polys begin to disappear after the second day unless infection is present, and when they die, polys release lysosomal enzymes that digest necrotic debris.

Multiple factors determine whether or not contaminating bacteria will proliferate to the point of infection (10^6 organisms/mm^3 for most pathogens) at a wound site. The amount of contamination and tissue destruction, the state of the circulation, and lymphatic drainage all play a role.

The initial presence of macrophages is proportional to the monocyte concentration in blood. Because the macrophage survives longer than the poly, it becomes the predominant WBC in the wound after the third day.

The macrophage disposes of necrotic tissue and foreign material. It also plays a critical part in initiating the next phase of healing by attracting fibroblasts

23

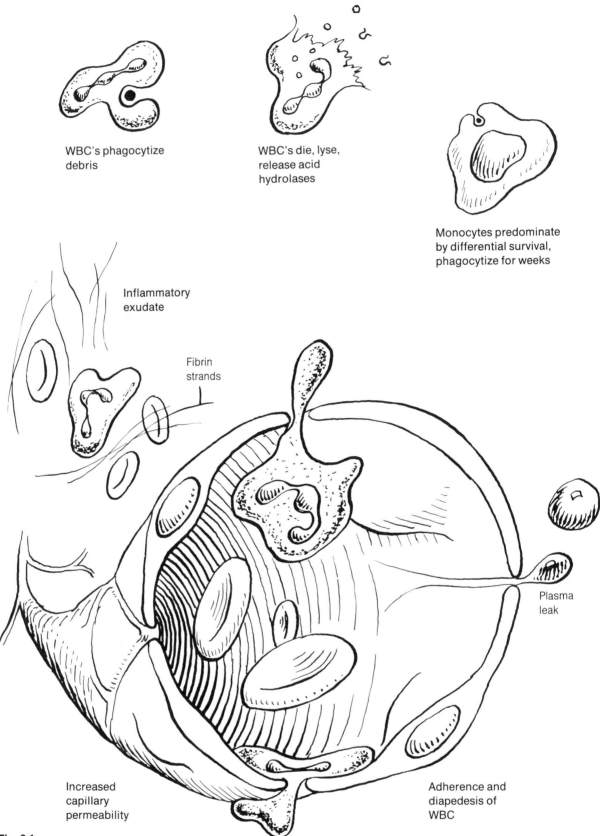

WBC's phagocytize
debris

WBC's die, lyse,
release acid
hydrolases

Monocytes predominate
by differential survival,
phagocytize for weeks

Inflammatory
exudate

Fibrin
strands

Plasma
leak

Increased
capillary
permeability

Adherence and
diapedesis of
WBC

Fig. 2.1

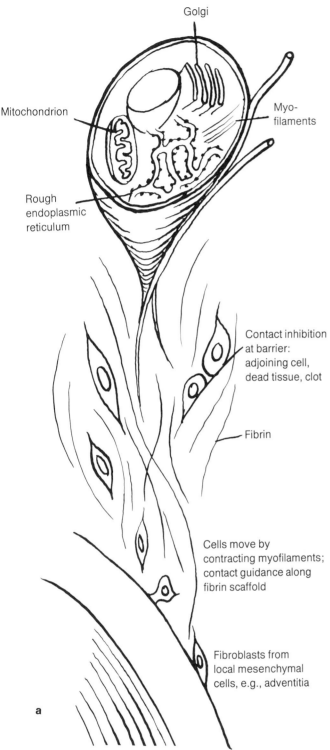

Golgi

Myo-filaments

Mitochondrion

Rough endoplasmic reticulum

Contact inhibition at barrier: adjoining cell, dead tissue, clot

Fibrin

Cells move by contracting myofilaments; contact guidance along fibrin scaffold

Fibroblasts from local mesenchymal cells, e.g., adventitia

a

wound but are attached through a binding protein, probably fibronectin. They move along the fibrin scaffolding with the aid of their contractile myofilaments. Their movement is limited by infection and contact inhibition at a barrier such as dead tissue. By the tenth day, fibroblasts are the predominant cells in the wound.

Epithelialization begins very early after wounding. By 24 hours the epidermis at the edge of the wound thickens, and marginal basal cells loosen, enlarge, and begin to migrate in the wound. Fixed basal cells divide rapidly to produce daughter cells that migrate along fibrin strands. In a primarily apposed wound, epithelialization can be complete by 48 hours. The epithelium and fibrin bridge are the only elements contributing to tensile strength at this stage.

Epithelium over scars is thinner and less firmly attached than normal. Its poor blood supply makes it vulnerable to pressure necrosis.

Endothelial cells migrate into the injured area from wounded vessels immediately after fibroblasts. These cells have a potent plasminogen activator that leads to fibrinolysis and destruction of the fibrin network. The result is an extensive new capillary network. The advancing capillaries move toward areas of low oxygen tension. Capillary budding and proliferation seem to be related to the prior invasion of macrophages. The fragile new capillaries are sensitive to changes in osmolarity and blood pressure (see Fig. 2.2).

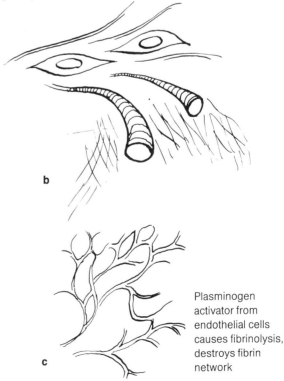

b

Plasminogen activator from endothelial cells causes fibrinolysis, destroys fibrin network

c

Fig. 2.2　a) Fibroblast, b) Collagen fibers (at 4–5 days), c) Rapid capillary proliferation

and influencing their maturation, division, and collagen synthesis.

Fibroblasts begin to appear as early as 24 hours after injury. These cells differentiate from local mesenchymal cells, mainly from adventitia. They do not attach directly to the collagen or fibrin in the

Fibroplasia

As necrotic tissue and debris are removed, fibroblast proliferation and migration are facilitated. When migrating epithelial cells and fibroblasts contact debris, they produce collagenase, which breaks down collagen.

Fibroblasts initially produce only ground substance, containing protein polysaccharides and glycoproteins. Significant collagen synthesis begins about the fourth day. Direction of fibroblast activity seems to be under the influence of the macrophage. The fibroblasts require nutrients and O_2 from the new capillaries. The capillaries in turn need collagen for support to contain the blood. Thus a delicate mutual dependence exists.

Collagen production rapidly increases over the next 2–4 weeks. The excess collagen laid down in this period is known as a healing ridge. At the end of this period, the number of fibroblasts begins to decrease and the rate of collagen synthesis declines. The capillary networks are reduced to a few well-defined systems.

At 4 weeks an equilibrium is reached between synthesis and destruction. Remodeling begins and proceeds for several months (see Fig. 2.3).

Collagen Synthesis

The stimulus that tells the fibroblast to differentiate and begin collagen synthesis is unknown. The earliest such mitogen may be the recently identified platelet-derived growth factor (PDGF) released by thrombin-activated platelets.

All of the five known types of collagen consist of three polypeptides (alpha chains) of equal length wrapped in a triple helix. Most of the alpha chain is helical and contains glycine in every third position (GLY-X-Y). Thus glycine constitutes 33% of the amino acid content of collagen. Collagen also has two unique amino acids, hydroxyproline and hydroxylysine, which occur only in the Y position.

Alpha-chain synthesis takes place on the ribosomes of the rough endoplasmic reticulum of the fibroblast. The alpha chains contain about 1000 amino acids and have nonhelical N-terminal and C-terminal telopeptide regions. During and shortly after synthesis, most proline and lysine residues are hydroxylated by enzymes that require Fe^{++}, O_2, α-ketoglutarate, and ascorbic acid as cofactors. Hydroxyproline plays important roles in formation and stabilization of the triple helix and in cross-linking, as does hydroxylysine. When the alpha chains are released into the cysternae of the endoplasmic reticulum, cysteine residues in the N-terminal telopeptide interact to form disulfide bonds linking three alpha chains together to form procollagen. Hydroxylation ends as the triple helix forms. The alignment of the helix allows further bonding of the helical regions of the molecules.

The procollagen is secreted into the extracellular space via the Golgi apparatus. There, cell membrane-bound proteases cleave off most of the N-terminal and C-terminal peptides *en bloc*. The resulting collagen molecule (also called tropocollagen) is a rigid rod $3,000 \times 15$ Å with a molecular weight of 270,000. The collagen is rapidly aggregated into a quarter-stagger array held by electrostatic forces. This arrangement results in the characteristic 640-Å banding seen in type I collagen. As progressively stronger types of bonds occur, the collagen loses its solubility in water, saline, and finally acid. This increase in bonding strength and fiber size is known as maturation.

Collagen Maturation

Around the time collagen molecules are being incorporated into fibers, another critical reaction is taking place. Oxidative deamination converts lysine to allysine and hydroxylysine to hydroxy-allysine. This prepares the way for covalent intra- and intermolecular cross-links by condensation of aldehydes. These are the bonds that give collagen its tensile strength.

Molecules must be less than 15 Å apart for cross-linking to occur, and therefore tight packing and possibly tension are important. The collagen fiber grows by accretion of new polymer chains and possibly surface aggregation of collagen molecules. As the fiber enlarges, the center becomes more compact and maximal cross-linking occurs there. Thus the center of the fiber becomes less soluble; the other layers are more susceptible to acids and neutral salts. Cross-linking continues after normal fiber size is reached.

Fig. 2.3

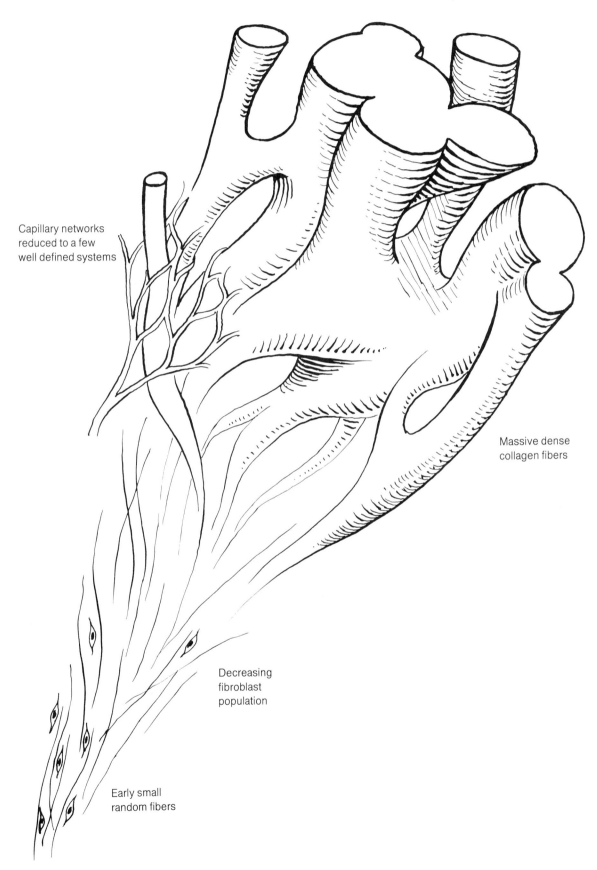

Remodeling over
many months

Capillary networks
reduced to a few
well defined systems

Massive dense
collagen fibers

Decreasing
fibroblast
population

Early small
random fibers

Remodeling

When collagen synthesis reaches an equilibrium with collagen destruction in a wound, strength gain depends on cross-linking and reorganization. Tissue collagenase – normally found in the upper dermis, in migrating epithelial cells, and in granulation tissue – attacks collagen at a specific site. The less stable fragments are denatured and then degraded by other proteases. Fibers oriented along lines of tension are preferentially spared. The more closely packed fibers have the greatest number of cross-links and are less susceptible to collagenase than peripheral random fibers. Thus there is progression from small, random fibers to larger, more organized fibers.

Because there is prolonged metabolic activity in scar tissue, anything that disturbs this balance – scurvy, for example – can lead to late scar breakdown.

Wound Strength

A wound's extensibility (the amount it will stretch before it breaks) is dependent on the nonelastic stretch of its strongest component, collagen; there are no elastin fibers in scar tissue. Cross-linking increases breaking strength, but at a certain point the scar tissue becomes brittle to shearing forces.

Tensile strength, defined as the load applied per unit cross-sectional area at the time of breaking, increases rapidly after the first week (during which the wound regains only about 5% of the original tissue strength). In the first several weeks, this increase is due to collagen synthesis; later gain in strength is due to increased cross-linking. The rate of gain in tensile strength varies from tissue to tissue; the maximum final strength is usually less than that of unwounded tissue.

Factors Affecting Healing

Various factors affect wound healing, including the etiology of the wound, delay of treatment, and age and health of the patient.

Infection is the most significant early deterrent to wound healing. A large inoculum of bacteria, necrotic tissue, a foreign body, or decreased host defense can contribute to the growth of pathogens beyond the control of local defense mechanisms.

Anything that compromises the local microcirculation has an adverse effect on healing and promotes infection. Hypovolemia, severe anemia, and low oxygen tension impair the body's ability to deliver oxygen and nutrients. Sludging associated with hypovolemia, low flow states, or hypothermia has the same effect. This type of local stasis and intravascular coagulation is common in trauma. The edema associated with injury can cause a snug suture to strangulate tissue. A pressure dressing also compromises local microcirculation. Obstructive vascular disease on either the gross level (atherosclerosis) or the microscopic level (diabetic microangiopathy, vasculitis) results in ischemic, nonhealing wounds. Poor circulation prevents antibiotics from reaching the wound. Wounds in areas of chronic venous stasis also heal poorly. Radiation endarteritis results in the destruction of local blood supply, making wounds in radiated areas notoriously slow to heal.

The circumstances surrounding the production of a wound have a direct impact on healing. A wound contaminated by fecal soilage will be much more prone to infection and sepsis than a relatively clean wound. Delay of treatment increases exposure time, tissue dessication, and infection risk. Massive trauma resulting in multiple organ injury impairs the body's ability to deal with each individual insult.

The preinjury health of a patient influences healing. Diabetes and uremia have profound negative effects on repair. Systemic diseases, especially such chronically debilitating processes as inflammatory bowel disease and cancer, can compromise the repair process.

General nutrition is important for protein anabolism (amino acid substrate, vitamin and mineral cofactors) and for host defense. Malnutrition is probably the cause of poor healing seen in jaundiced patients. Anergy associated with malnutrition is a reflection of decreased immune competence and decreased resistance to infection.

Steroids and other anti-inflammatory and cytotoxic drugs can have an adverse effect on wound healing.

Specific agents inhibit collagen synthesis and maturation. Proline analogues inhibit helix formation, β-Aminoproprionitrile and D-penicillamine both inhibit cross-linking: the former by inhibiting lysyl oxidase, the latter by binding to aldehydes. Such agents may prove useful in controlling unwanted fibrosis, e.g., around cut nerves and tendons or in cirrhosis.

Practical Considerations

Immediately after injury, careful physiological monitoring allows early treatment of fluid, electrolyte, and ventilatory derangement. Irreversible damage to the microcirculation can thus be avoided and the risk of infection is decreased.

Minimal movement and talking in the operating room help decrease dissemination of airborne bacteria, the major source of exogenous contamination. Having the patient shower with antiseptic soap before surgery and shaving the operative area immediately prior to surgery further decrease the chance of contamination.

Wounds subject to a high infection risk should be left open to granulate for about 4 days. Granulation tissue is highly resistant to infection. The wound may then be closed secondarily.

Gentle tissue handling, careful hemostasis, thorough debridement, and careful sterile technique in surgery decrease the risk of infection and promote healing. Efficient surgery is also beneficial, since the rate of contamination increases dramatically after prolonged tissue exposure. Antibiotics should be used when appropriate.

Nutritional support with parenteral alimentation has been a major benefit to seriously injured and debilitated patients for the reasons discussed above. Systemic and local disease processes should be effectively treated at all times.

Fine suture material or tape causes the least trauma to tissue at the wound edge. Any suture material, no matter how inert, carries a greater infection risk than tape. Sutures in structures expected to remain viable should be tied just snugly enough to loosely approximate edges. The edema that inevitably follows wounding will cause tight sutures to strangulate tissue and cut through. Extremity wounds should be elevated postoperatively to reduce edema.

A potential cause of dehiscence is placing sutures too close to the cut edge. The collagen breakdown accompanying the repair process weakens the tissue adjacent to the wound edge and may cause narrow bites to cut through.

Scar tissue feels hard and resists needle penetration, but it is brittle and lacks the strength of normal tissue. Suturing scar tissue to scar tissue is a risky proposition and probably accounts for the increased incidence of recurrence following secondary hernia repair. If one cannot find normal tissue to suture, it is sometimes preferable to excise scar tissue and bridge the gap with prosthetic material.

The time for safe suture removal varies from one area of the body to another. Healing is most rapid in the face and neck, where sutures may be removed as early as the second day. On the extremities, it may be necessary to wait as long as 2 weeks. Sutures on the trunk are safely removed after 1 week. To avoid suture marks, one can replace alternate sutures with tape earlier than the above times. The first tapes maintain tension as the remaining sutures are replaced. The presence of a healing ridge is a good indication that wound repair is progressing normally. However, don't mistake the tender swelling of a wound abscess for a healing ridge.

Summary

At the edge of a wound, cells have been killed and more cells are dying from dessication and loss of blood supply. Foreign material and bacteria combined with the dead tissue, serum, and blood pose a risk of infection. An active repair process requiring increased metabolic support must go on at a time when the supply lines are cut and blocked. The surgeon's task is to support the repair process and not add to the existing handicaps.

The surgeon does this by treating systemic diseases and nutritional defects and by monitoring and correcting volume, ventilatory, and chemical defects. The final and most important element is that over which the surgeon has the most control: the practice of good surgical technique, as described in the following section.

Surgical Technique, Wound Management, and Skin Grafting

Although there are no known ways to "accelerate" wound healing or to bypass the orderly sequence of events just discussed, the surgeon *can* promote early healing by removing obstacles to the healing process. In elective operations this involves planning the incision for optimal exposure, handling tissues properly, and utilizing operating time as efficiently as possible. The result is a reduction of iatrogenic tissue injury, a decrease of fluid loss through evaporation, decreased tissue drying, and decreased exposure to bacteria. In trauma cases obstacles to healing can be eliminated by thorough debridement and timely wound closure.

Necrotic debris (including charred tissue from the electrocautery) and foreign bodies (including suture material) are negative influences on the healing process since they must be cleared away by phagocytic cells before healing can begin. In traumatic wounds the effects of surgery are superimposed on tissues that are already compromised.

Elective Incisions

An ample incision that provides generous exposure is necessary for a safe operation. The incision should take into account adjacent neurovascular structures so they can be avoided or gently retracted. Such planning can prevent injuries that cause postoperative numbness and hypesthesias. The two goals of planning the incision are to provide safe access to underlying structures and to leave a reasonably cosmetic scar, with emphasis on the former.

In the head and neck region, the thin muscles that animate the face are intimately connected to the undersurface of the skin (Fig. 2.4). These cause the

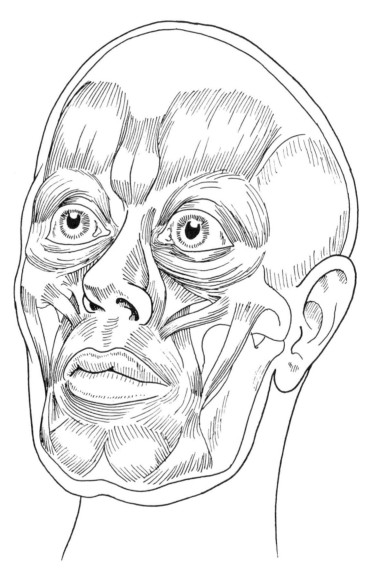

Fig. 2.4   The muscles of facial expression are intimately connected to the undersurface of the skin.

skin to wrinkle or "gather" in a predictable fashion perpendicular to the direction of muscle contraction (Fig. 2.5). For example, when the frontalis musculoaponeurotic sheet contracts, it pulls the eyebrows cephalad and gathers up the overlying forehead skin into transverse furrows. If one places an incision within or parallel to one of these furrows, it will be somewhat concealed by the "natural wrinkles." In addition, there will be less tension on the incision, since activation of the underlying muscle tends to close the wound rather than pull it apart.

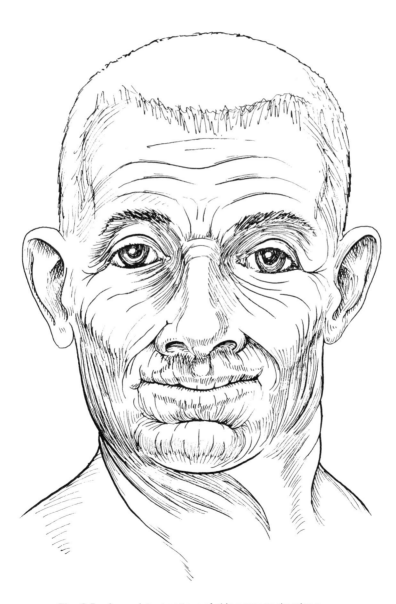

Fig. 2.5   A consistent pattern of skin creases develops perpendicular to the pull of the underlying muscles. Incisions parallel to these creases are less noticeable.

Another principle that has been applied to facial surgery is the concept of "aesthetic units." If it is necessary to excise large areas of facial skin, it is better to excise an entire "unit" and to reconstruct the defect with a single skin graft or tissue flap than it is to excise only a portion of that unit (Fig. 2.6). In this way, the final result will be concealed much more effectively and cosmetically. Incisions can also be planned so that they are on the borderlines of adjacent aesthetic units (such as the nasolabial fold). The resulting scars are much less noticeable than if they run counter to these units. Some authors subdivide these units into even smaller areas.

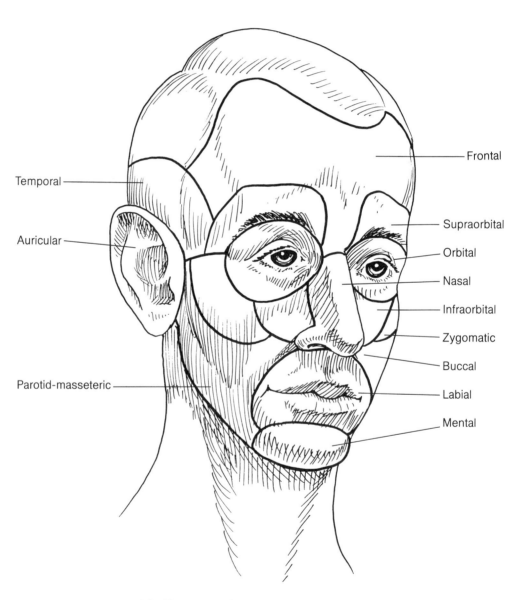

Fig. 2.6   The concept of aesthetic units defines facial skin areas that should be totally rather than partially replaced.

The standard chest wall incisions are the midline sternotomy and the posterolateral thoracotomy (Fig. 2.7). The sternotomy allows excellent access to the heart and mediastinal structures and, since it avoids neurovascular bundles, leaves the patient surprisingly free of pain. The posterolateral thoracotomy is usually made just above or in the bed of the fifth rib and avoids the major intercostal nerves. On the abdomen the midline incision provides excellent access to virtually all intraperitoneal structures and has the same virtues as the median sternotomy. Other abdominal incisions may be equally effective, and the choice is often based on the diagnosis and the preference of the surgeon. The primary concern in closing the chest or abdomen is the repair of the musculoskeletal layer.

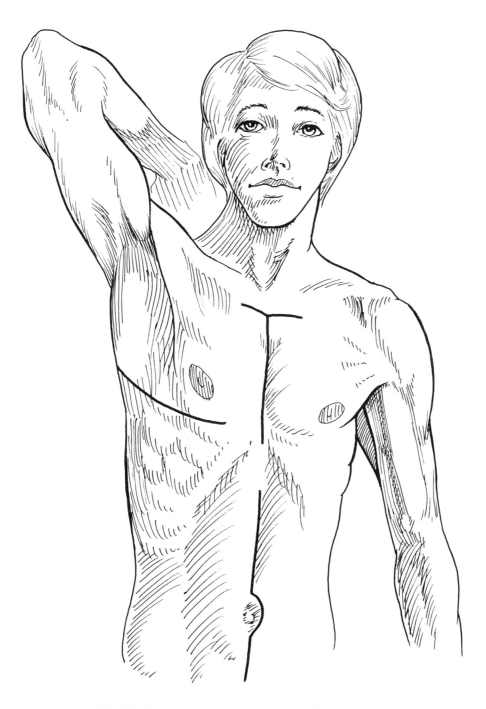

Fig. 2.7 Incisions such as the sternotomy, lateral thoracotomy, and midline abdominal incision cause minimal pain because they lie between neural territories.

Extremity incisions are usually made in an axial direction over the long bones. These give excellent exposure while avoiding cutaneous nerves (Fig. 2.8). The tissues are also easier to approximate in this direction. Over the flexor aspect of joints, the incision should curve and follow the flexion crease for several centimeters or as long as possible (Fig. 2.9). Incisions that cross such a flexion crease in an axial direction usually result in a web (due to the forces of natural wound contraction), which can limit full extension of the joint. Over the extensor aspect of a joint, a paramedian axial incision usually provides excellent and safe exposure (Fig. 2.10).

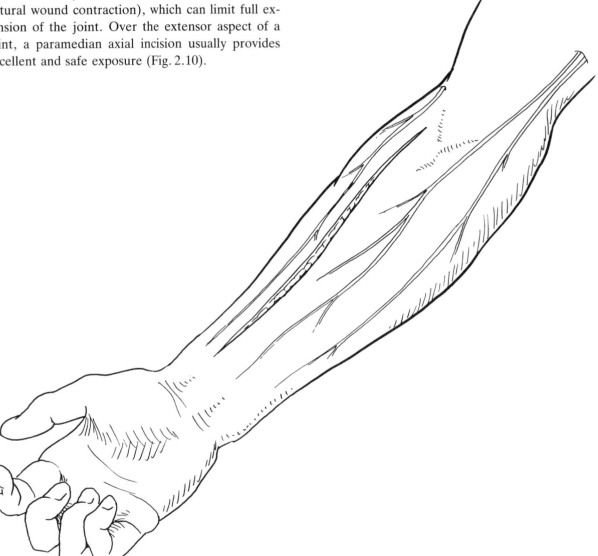

Fig. 2.8   Axial extremity incisions cause the least damage to cutaneous nerves.

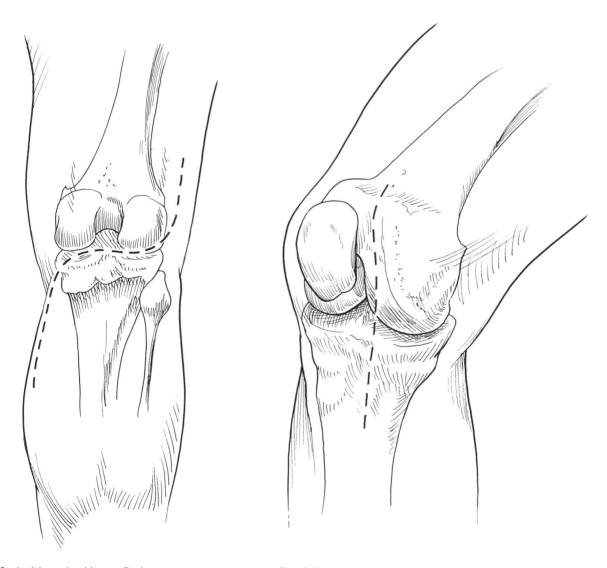

Fig. 2.9   Incisions should cross flexion creases transversely to prevent weblike contractions that can limit extension.

Fig. 2.10   Longitudinal incisions are appropriate on the extensor side of joints.

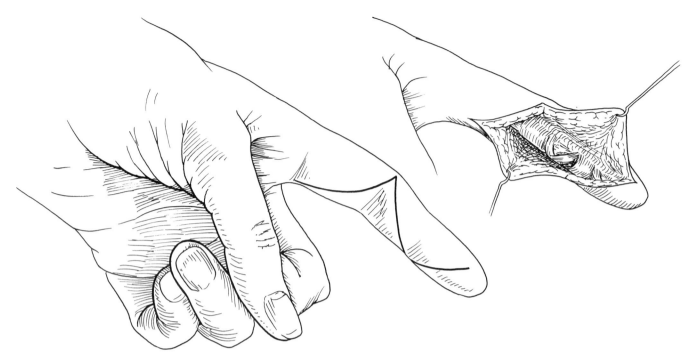

Fig. 2.11   The zig-zag incision gives good exposure of the volar aspect of the finger without compromising the flexion creases.

In the hand, incisions are designed to preserve the interdigital web spaces and the skin over the joints, especially on the palmar aspect. Many elaborate designs have been used. One of the easiest is the zig-zag or Bruner incision (Fig. 2.11). On the extensor side a straight axial incision gives excellent exposure (Fig. 2.12).

Fig. 2.12   An axial incision provides good exposure of the extensor side of the finger.

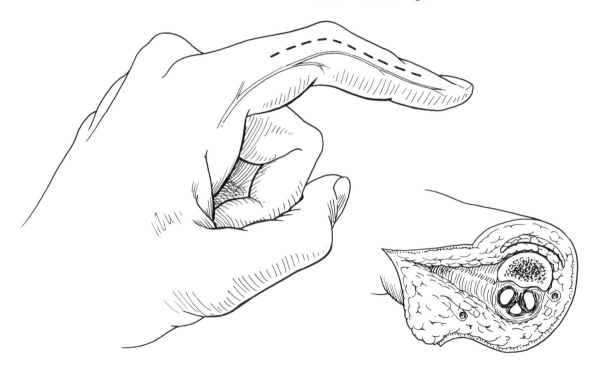

Trauma, Wound Management, and Skin Grafting

The lacerated edges of a traumatic wound should be conservatively excised, and any obviously nonviable tissue must be sharply removed from the depths of the wound (Fig. 2.13, a and b). Only after thorough debridement should one use irrigation or jet lavage to clear away the residual debris. Such irrigation is largely ineffective for small particulate matter such as dirt. The water stream serves only to make the particles vibrate within the tissue rather than exit the wound. These particles must be removed sharply.

Wounds in which there has been significant bacterial contamination are best left open and packed with sterile sponges after the initial debridement (Fig. 2.13c). The packing is kept moist with sterile saline to prevent desiccation of the tissues, and the

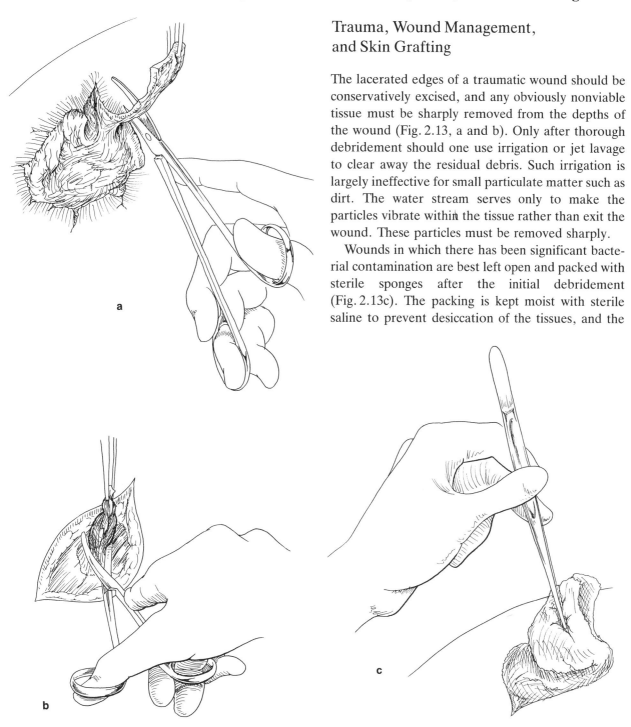

Fig. 2.13 The edges of a traumatic wound should be conservatively trimmed (a). Nonviable tissue is sharply excised from the depth of the wound (b). The wound is left open and packed with sterile sponges (c).

wound is reinspected 48–72 hours later under aseptic conditions. A clean appearance at that time correlates well with a bacterial count of less than 10^6 organisms per gram of tissue, and the wound can be closed with little risk of infection. A wound covered with exudate, on the other hand, indicates significant bacterial contamination. That wound is not ready for closure and must be debrided again. The cycle is repeated until healthy granulation tissue forms and the wound is clear of exudate. It can then be closed by approximating the wound edges or by the application of a skin graft. It is important that such grafts be "meshed" (see Fig. 2.14 and accompanying text).

When contaminated wounds are packed open for later closure, healing time is not lost. No significant collagen synthesis occurs in the wound for the first few days, and if the wound is closed secondarily at the end of this physiological lag period, healing will proceed at the same rate as a primarily closed clean wound. By closing a dirty wound primarily, one runs a great risk of deep abscess formation and unnecessary destruction of adjacent tissue by invasive pathogenic bacteria. Life-threatening septicemia may result. This can be avoided by conservative and judicious care of the contaminated wound and by not succumbing to an overwhelming urgency to close the wound too early.

If a wound must be left open for more than five to seven days because of lingering contamination or infection, the adjacent soft tissues lose their pliability from the effects of inflammation and edema. The chronic exposure makes the wound friable and effaces the soft tissue planes in the area. As a result such wounds are difficult to close by the mobilization of adjacent tissues. Indeed, such mobilization often leads to shredding of tissues and increased bleeding from the extensive vascular network that is present to support the metabolic demands of wound healing. It is often best, under these circumstances, to use a skin graft to close the wound. This will allow the wound to heal rapidly and avoid the chronic changes of an open wound that lead to edema and fibrosis. The skin-grafted wound will soften rapidly, and if deemed necessary, the graft can be excised later, and the tissues can be mobilized to provide a more natural contour.

When there has been loss of skin, the same principles apply. After the initial debridement the wound is packed open with sterile sponges that are kept moist with normal saline solution. After 48–72 hours have elapsed, the wound is examined, using aseptic technique. If the wound appears clean at that time, a split-thickness skin graft can be applied to provide the closure. The safest closure for such open wounds is with a meshed, split-thickness skin graft (Fig. 2.14). However, there are a few technical points which should be noted.

A split-thickness skin graft relies on the ingrowth of new capillaries from the underlying granulation tissue for survival. Three major factors can disrupt this process and cause graft failure: movement of the graft, fluid beneath the graft, and infection. Stability is achieved by suturing the graft at multiple points and by applying a secure dressing. The latter two problems are avoided by meshing the graft. The interstices allow free drainage of the fluid that invariably weeps from the underlying raw surface. The evacuation of such fluid removes the culture medium that predisposes wounds to bacterial growth. When such a wound does become infected, β-hemolytic streptococcus is usually the organism responsible. For this reason all grafts should be protected for approximately 72 hours with prophylactic systemic penicillin or another antibiotic to which the streptococcus organism is susceptible.

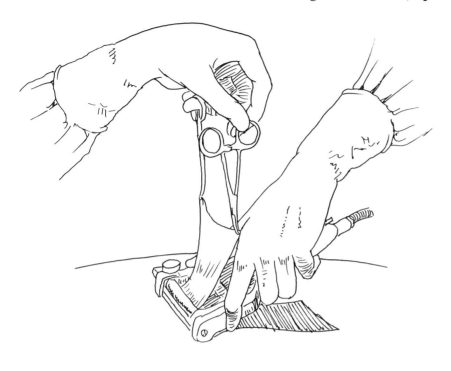

Fig. 2.14   The meshed, split-thickness skin graft provides safe, rapid cover for a clean open wound.

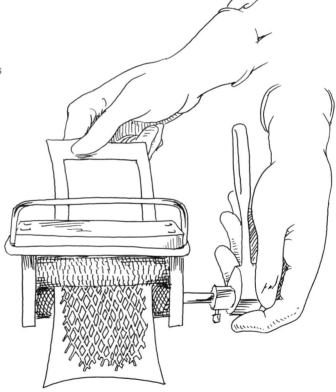

Chapter 3

Surgical Knots
and Suture Materials

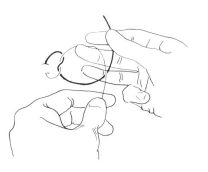

Introduction

Tying surgical knots can be simple and straightforward to learn and practice if basic principles are followed. The square knot (also called a reef knot, true knot, or sailor's knot) should be learned well and may be used exclusively. Variations and combinations may be tried later. In most surgeons' hands the two-handed knot is more precise, although it takes slightly longer to perform than the one-handed knot. One will never be criticized for using the two-handed tie.

The strand that is actively passed through the loop will be designated the "working" strand in the following descriptions. By choosing the appropriate end for your working strand and using the appropriate throw first, it should never be necessary to cross your strands or hands.

A distinction must be made between a half knot and a half hitch. The former is a single flat throw that constitutes half of a square or half of a granny (false) knot. The half hitch is a single throw in which one strand is looped around the other, taut strand, thus forming a slip knot. The most common error in knot tying is not maintaining equal tension on the strands and thereby converting a flat half knot into a sliding half hitch.

The following diagrams teach all knots with the right hand manipulating the working strand, since most people are right-handed. The left-handed surgeon (or the right-handed surgeon who would like to learn a left-handed one-hand knot) should study the diagrams in a mirror.

Once the basic knots are mastered, it is a simple matter to apply tension or tie in a difficult location.

41

Basic Principles

1. The working strand is always manipulated by the right hand (the left-handed person may find it easier to master the knots described here by studying the following diagrams in the mirror). At the conclusion of each throw, the strands have reversed their starting position.

2. Measure a comfortable length of suture so that you are not cramped and there is no great redundancy. The hands should be equidistant from the site of the knot. Both the right and left hands must grasp their respective strands at a point that allows the tip of the outstretched index finger to just reach the knot (see Figs. 3.1–3.4).

3. Choose the appropriate first throw so that neither the suture nor your hands will cross. The proper first throw is easily determined by deciding whether the strand held by the left hand (nonworking end) is toward or away from you (see Figs. 3.5–3.8).

4. Don't be afraid to turn your body so that your hands are oriented properly. Visualize your knots as being tied toward or away from your body and you will virtually eliminate crossing.

5. Keep the strands loose and equal, forming a round loop as you snug the knot down. This will prevent formation of a half hitch and prevent sawing and fraying. This also avoids disturbing the first throw.

6. Alternate throws to form a square knot. Repeating the same throw results in a granny knot.

7. Learn to complete the throw by putting the index finger of the hand holding the strand (whether it is your left or right) closest to your body down on the knot. This finger thus is below (dependent to) the knot. This prevents pulling up on structures you are tying and prevents reversing the throw into a half hitch.

8. Approximate tissue, don't strangulate it.

9. A slight jiggle at the end of each throw will help tighten one throw on top of another.

As in learning any other skill, repetitious practice is essential to making the process automatic. Practice combined with these principles will allow you to tie efficient, accurate, and secure knots.

The middle, ring, and little finger of each hand grasp the respective strands at a distance that places the index finger at the knot.

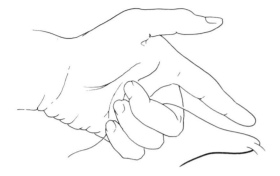

Fig. 3.1 The grasp on the strand held by the left hand never changes. The strand initially held by the left hand determines the set-up of the first throw (see Figs. 3.5–3.8).

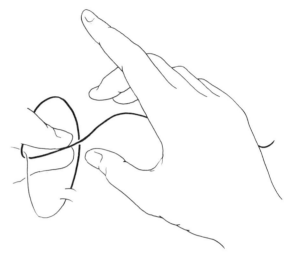

Fig. 3.3 The right hand must repeatedly regrasp the working strand. The same distance rule applies.

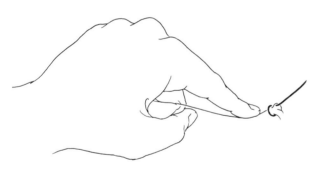

Fig. 3.2 The left index finger is placed down on the knot when the strand held by the left hand (nonworking strand) finishes the throw toward the operator.

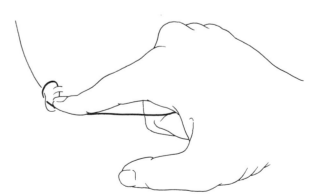

Fig. 3.4 When the working strand finishes the throw toward the operator, the right index fingertip goes down on the knot.

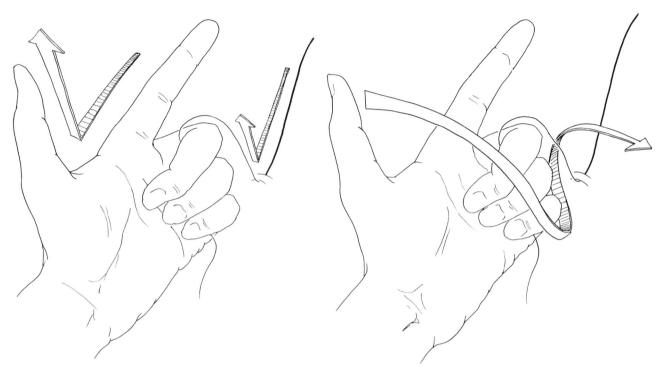

Fig. 3.5 The "V" formed by the thumb and index fingers of the left hand can be thought of as corresponding to the "V" formed by the strands. When the nonworking strand is toward the operator, the thumb, which is also toward the operator, sets up the throw.

Fig. 3.6 The finger (the thumb in this case) that sets up the throw is always passed between the strands from left to right. Proceed from Fig. 3.15.

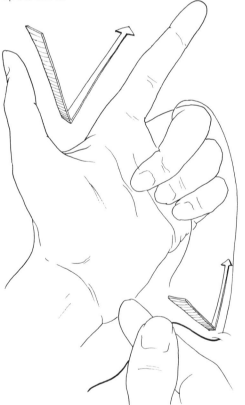

Fig. 3.7 When the working strand starts away from the operator, the left index finger, which is also away from operator, sets up the throw.

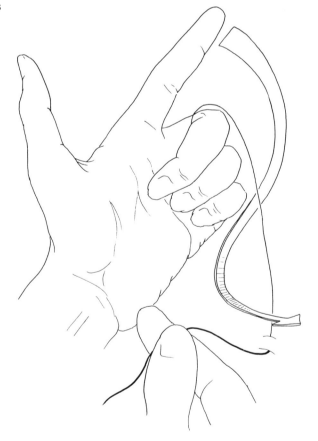

Fig. 3.8 The index finger is passed between the strands from left to right, ending in a position that is perpendicular to the plane of the loop that is formed next (see Fig. 3.9).

The Knots

In the following illustrations (Fig. 3.9–3.35), the knots are shown only partially tightened, for the purpose of clarity. The working strand is shown by the heavier line.

Note that the first step for every throw is the formation of a loop over a finger or instrument and that the strands between the structure being tied and the finger are never crossed. Keeping the finger parallel to the structure (incision, vessel) being tied prevents twisting of the loop and crossing.

Either throw may be used first in any knot, depending on which strand is most convenient to use as the working end (e.g., the end without the needle). Tie enough alternating throws to create a secure knot with the suture material used.

To achieve optimal snugness without breaking the strand, a series of quick, short pulls or "jiggle" is much more effective than a steady force. The latter is often referred to as "the jerk at the end of the tie," especially when the strand breaks. A properly tightened throw will usually remain in place if it is not disturbed in creating the next throw. Occasionally separation of wound edges may necessitate a friction knot or a "tension tie."

If it seems necessary to tie with tension, it may mean that the dissection is inadequate to allow easy edge approximation. Such circumstances lead to tissue necrosis and the stitches cutting through in a short time.

The preferred length for an individual ligature or "free tie" varies among surgeons. An 18-inch length comfortably makes two knots. Longer strands of suture material are available on a spool or reel that is held in the left hand and feeds the material as needed for multiple ties.

When a suture material is used in the procedures in Part II, a common choice of type and diameter for that purpose is noted.

The orientation shown here – tying toward and away from the operator – is a constructive departure from the traditional teaching of surgical knots. The throws shown for creating the two-hand knot are standard. The throws presented for the one-hand method are chosen from the three commonly used variants (the throw not shown is the alternate method for starting with the working strand away from the operator).

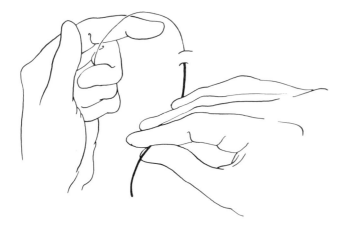

Fig. 3.9   The left index finger is in position to set up the loop.

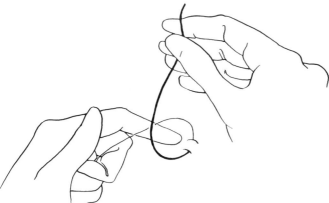

Fig. 3.10   Form a loop over the index finger, using the working strand in the right hand.

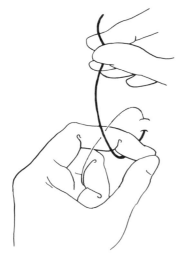

Fig. 3.11   Pinch left thumb and index finger together away from the intersecting strands of the loop.

To make a surgeon's or friction knot, repeat the steps shown in Figs. 3.11 through 3.13 to pass the working strand through the first loop two times.

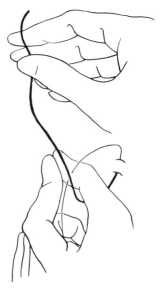

Fig. 3.12   Swing thumb and index finger to the opposite side of the loop to grasp the working strand. Shift the right shoulder in toward the table to make this move comfortably.

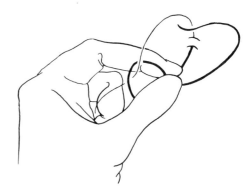

Fig. 3.13   Pass the working strand cleanly through the loop and regrasp it with the right hand, as in Fig. 3.3.

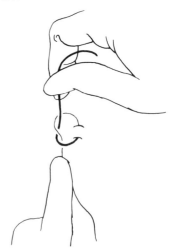

Fig. 3.14   The left index finger is now in proper position to put down next to the knot as the working strand is pulled to the side opposite the operator. The strands and knot are kept in a straight line each time a throw is tightened.

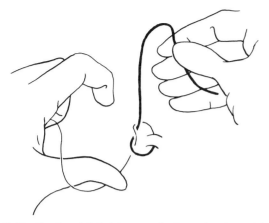

Fig. 3.15 The thumb is held perpendicular to the plane of the strands.

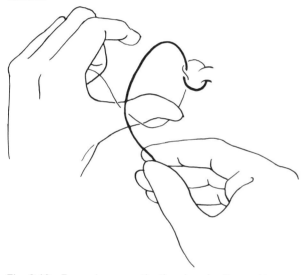

Fig. 3.16 Form a loop over the thumb, using the working strand in the right hand.

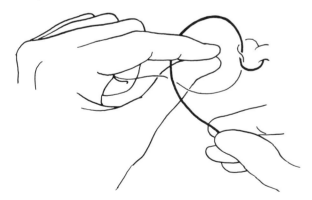

Fig. 3.17 Pinch left thumb and index finger together, keeping clear of the loop.

In the two-hand tie the left hand takes an active part in setting up the loop and manipulating the working strand. It is important to do the pinching maneuvers away from the loop to avoid entanglement.

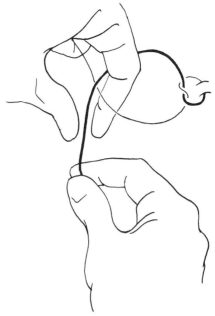

Fig. 3.18 Swing thumb and index finger to the opposite side of the loop to grasp the working strand. Rotate the left shoulder in toward the patient at this point.

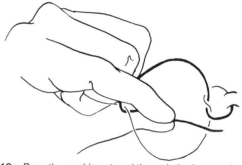

Fig. 3.19 Pass the working strand through the loop and regrasp it with the right hand, as in Fig. 3.3.

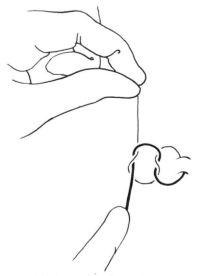

Fig. 3.20 The right index finger is now in proper position to put down next to the knot as the working strand is pulled toward the operator. For either throw the opposite index finger may also be pronated on its strand for added precision.

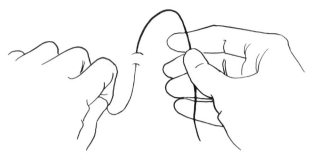

Fig. 3.21 Drape a comfortable length of working strand over the fingers of the right hand, grasping the strand with the thumb and middle fingers.

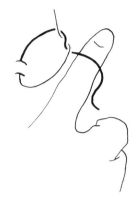

Fig. 3.24 Sweep the working strand through the loop with the index finger.

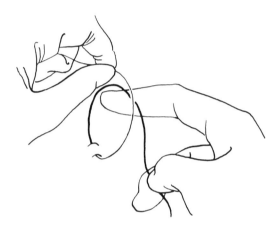

Fig. 3.22 Move the nonworking strand over the right index finger to set up a loop.

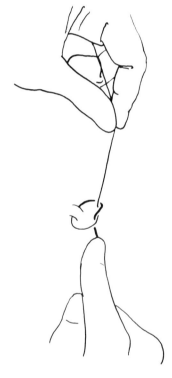

Fig. 3.25 Grasp the working strand with the right hand and tighten with the right index finger.

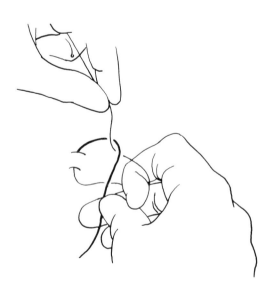

Fig. 3.23 Flex the right index finger, catching the nonworking strand.

Note that the working strand has finished opposite to where it started. Keeping a smooth open loop until the throw is tight helps keep this key relationship clear. It also prevents reversing the throw into a half hitch, which happens more frequently with the one-hand tie. If the left (or nondependent) index finger were placed below the knot, the throw would be reversed into a half hitch.

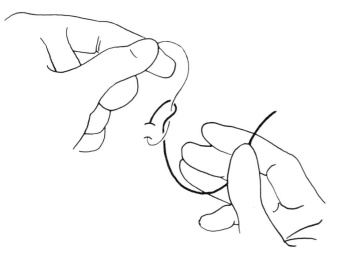

Fig. 3.26 Drape the working strand over the fingers of the right hand from the ulnar side, with the thumb and index finger grasping the strand.

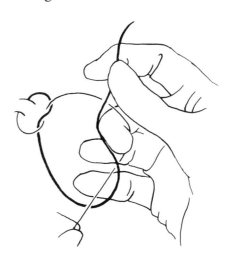

Fig. 3.28 Flex the middle finger to pull the nonworking strand behind the working strand.

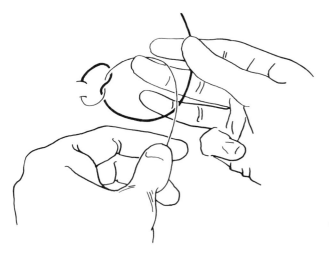

Fig. 3.27 Move the nonworking strand over the right middle finger to set up a loop.

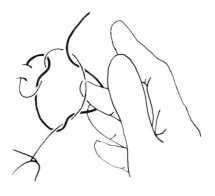

Fig. 3.29 Sweep the working strand through the loop, using the right middle finger.

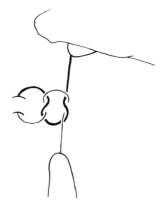

In the one-hand tie the right hand sets up the loop and manipulates the working strand. Compare this to the two-hand tie.

Fig. 3.30 Tighten the throw with the left index finger.

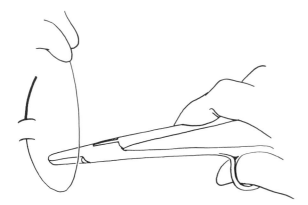

Fig. 3.31   Hold the needle-holder parallel with the incision or vessel being tied. Drape the nonworking end over the instrument. Leave the working end short.

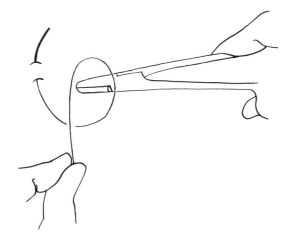

Fig. 3.32   Form a loop around the instrument. Make a double loop if a friction knot is desired.

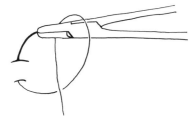

Fig. 3.33   Grasp the end of the working strand.

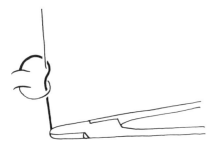

Fig. 3.34   Reverse the nonworking strand and bring the working end toward you.

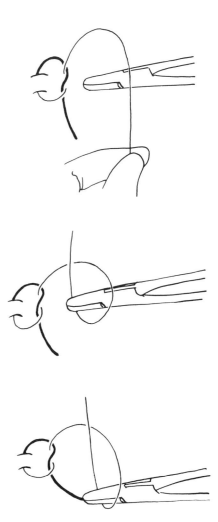

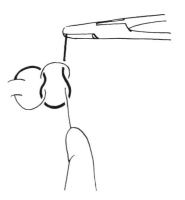

Fig. 3.35   Repeat the first four maneuvers shown in the left column in the opposite direction.

This tie is useful when working with very fine suture material and when multiple knots are needed, e.g., as in tacking down a skin graft. The needle-holder need not be held rigidly perpendicular to the axis of the loop but will move naturally to assist formation of the loop as you get a feel for this tie.

Suture Materials

The proliferation of synthetic suture materials in recent years has been accompanied by claims of superiority over other materials, but little objective critical evaluation has been done. Some recent studies, cited in the selected readings section, point out the questions that need to be answered.

Sutures are placed to hold tissues together; healing restores the wound to about 5% of the strength of the unwounded tissue in the first week. The additional gain in strength needed to make the support of suture material superfluous depends on the location. For long-term strength a permanent, nonabsorbable suture material is called for. For short-term use, an absorbable material is appropriate. The rate of reabsorption must correspond with the rate of healing.

The security of a suture depends on its intrinsic tensile strength and its ability to hold a knot. A suture or ligature fails either because the material breaks or because the knot slips. Both occur as a result of the strain on the material. It takes significant force to break the suture material. However, if the knot has the potential to slip, it does so at a much lower level of tension. The studies mentioned above consider both breakage and slippage as causes of knot failure. When breakage occurs, it invariably does so at the knot and is considered knot failure. Breakage is inversely proportional to tensile strength and diameter for all suture materials.

The second mechanism, knot slippage, is subject to more variables than is breakage. The security of knots tied by different surgeons varies. There is even variability among knots tied by the same individual. A suture material with a higher coefficient of friction has less tendency to slip. The type of knot, the number of turns per throw, and the number of throws per knot influence slippage. Flat throws are critical. A knot that ends as a double half hitch – regardless of whether it started as a square or granny – is a slip knot and has no holding power. The creation of a slip knot is more likely with one-hand ties.

Another consideration in choosing a suture material is its interaction with tissues. Some materials stimulate an intense inflammatory reaction (e.g., catgut) and others (e.g., wire) are almost totally inert. The higher coefficient of friction of braided materials helps hold knots but makes the suture harder to drag through tissue and thus more traumatic. In addition, braided materials have interstices that can harbor bacteria and act as wicks for capillary action.

Subcuticular nonabsorbable braided suture materials have been associated with diminished wound-breaking strength in dogs, probably because of the higher infection rate. The suture must be viewed as a foreign body. In order to leave minimal foreign material in the wound, it is desirable that a suture material have a high tensile strength at a small diameter. A high knot-holding capacity decreases the number of turns and throws necessary to form the minimum secure knot for a material. Halsted pointed out that a suture ligature permitted the use of finer suture material than would be necessary if the vessel were not transfixed (see Fig. 5.82).

A final consideration is the handling characteristics of material. Silk has long been the standard for excellent handling. Wire, at the other end of the spectrum, is capable of cutting the surgeon's hands.

Below is a list of the commonly used categories of suture materials. Cotton, linen, and metals besides stainless steel have been omitted. In the interest of clarity, the numerous brand names and varieties are not listed. The list is followed by a discussion of the properties of the suture materials in each group.

Natural suture materials
  Absorbable
    catgut (plain, chromic)
  Nonabsorbable
    silk

Synthetic suture materials
  Absorbable (polyesters)
    polyglycolic acid
    polyglactin 910
    polydioxanone

  Nonabsorbable (polyester, plastics)
    Dacron polyester
    nylon
    polypropylene
    polyethylene
    polybutester
    polytetrafluoroethylene

Stainless steel wire

When an absorbable suture material is required, the choice is between catgut and one of the newer polyesters. Two of these polyesters, polyglycolic acid and polyglactin 910, are braided, and one, polydioxanone, is a monofilament. Catgut is made from the collagenous submucosa of sheep intestine. Plain catgut elicits a marked foreign-body response and is rapidly absorbed ($\sim$ 10 days). By treating the surface of catgut with chromic acid, the inflammatory response of the body is retarded, absorption is slowed, and the tensile strength is maintained longer ($\sim$ 21 days). Catgut exhibits excellent knot security and freedom from slippage when dry. However, when it is wet, tensile strength decreases and knot security drops drastically. The tails of catgut must be cut long (¼ inch) to account for slippage. Other suture materials are minimally affected by wetting.

The synthetic absorbable materials have some advantage over catgut in that they are absorbed without significant tissue reaction. Also, the braided synthetic absorbable materials have a greater knot-holding ability because of their higher coefficient of friction. The newest synthetic absorbable suture, polydioxanone, maintains its tensile strength significantly longer than gut and other polyesters.

Silk is commonly used because of tradition, training, and individual preference for its excellent handling properties. In terms of tensile strength and knot-holding ability, silk compares poorly to some of the newer synthetics.

Dacron polyester is the strongest nonabsorbable material (excepting stainless steel wire). It has excellent knot security but suffers from the disadvantages of braided materials and does not handle as well as silk. Dacron is made coated with Teflon and coated or impregnated with silicone to overcome these disadvantages, but these forms show a markedly decreased knot security.

The monofilament plastics are unreactive and pull easily through tissue. They have intermediate tensile strength and only fair knot security, requiring several flat throws. Most are stiff and handle poorly. The newest monofilament, polybutester, is more flexible and elastic and may overcome these problems. There is a braided nylon available.

Another new nonabsorbable suture material, expanded polytetrafluoroethylene (PTFE), is something of a hybrid. Although not a true monofilament in view of its interstices, it is strong relative to the monofilaments and has comparable knot security. Its pliability gives it superior handling qualities.

Stainless steel wire is the strongest, least reactive, most secure suture material available. It is also the hardest to work with and the most traumatic to the surgeon's hands. Subcutaneous wire knots sometimes cause discomfort to the patient. Wire sutures that are twisted together rather than tied have negligible knot security.

There are few definite conclusions to be drawn from the available studies regarding knots. The most important observation is that any surgical knot must be completed with snug, flat throws. The advantage of the square knot over the granny knot is not clear cut. If either knot is turned into a double half hitch by unequal tension in tying, it is useless. The number of turns and number of throws are proportional in a general way to knot security. However, a material requiring multiple knots creates a larger foreign body.

There is no one suture that is optimal for all situations. The best the surgeon can do is make an educated choice.

Conclusion

It takes a combination of flat throws to create a secure knot. The two-handed square knot is the preferred surgical knot and should be learned well before variations are attempted. A minimum of three flat throws is made to complete a knot. Knot-holding ability depends on suture size, the nature of the suture material (tensile strength, surface friction), and the type and number of throws. Some suture materials, particularly coated materials and the synthetic monofilaments, require multiple throws for a secure knot. An additional turn within a throw (friction knot) may enhance holding power in some situations.

Sometimes an absorbable or nonabsorbable suture must be used for a particular purpose. When strength requirements exceed the capacity of an absorbable suture, dehiscence will result. When long-term suture strength is necessary (as in a vascular anastomosis), a permanent material such as polypropylene is appropriate. Other situations demand an absorbable suture, such as in the biliary and genitourinary systems where permanent sutures act as a nidus around which stones can grow.

The surgeon's goal is to choose the proper suture material for the job and the proper knot for the suture material.

Chapter 4

Instruments

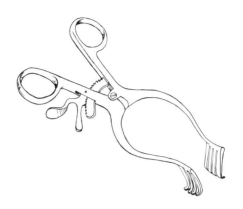

"All instruments ought to be well suited for the purpose in hand as regards their size, weight, and delicacy."

HIPPOCRATES (460–380 B.C.)

Instruments extend the capability of the surgeon's hands. Cutting and grasping instruments do the work of surgery; retractors and suction tips provide exposure. There are many variations of each instrument and numerous eponyms. Representative instruments in each category are illustrated in the following pages. Descriptive names are used whenever possible. Electrosurgical tools are discussed in the next chapter.

There are many highly specialized instruments used in surgical specialities. Miniaturization permits microsurgical techniques in ophthalmological and vascular surgery. Modifications that permit a longer reach are essential to otolaryngologists and neurosurgeons. Gentleness and delicacy characterize many vascular and cardiothoracic instruments. On the other hand, strength and power are often needed in orthopedics.

However exotic, most of these tools are but variations of the basic instruments.

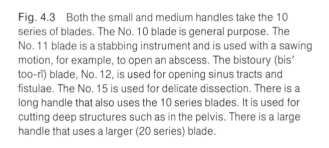

Fig. 4.1   A *small scalpel handle* is used for delicate dissection.

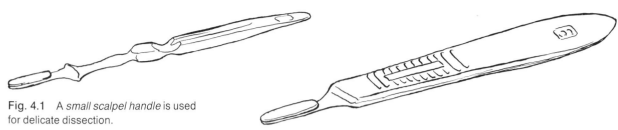

Fig. 4.2   The *medium scalpel handle* is used for almost all purposes. When the surgeon says "Knife," he usually wants this instrument.

Fig. 4.3   Both the small and medium handles take the 10 series of blades. The No. 10 blade is general purpose. The No. 11 blade is a stabbing instrument and is used with a sawing motion, for example, to open an abscess. The bistoury (bis' too-rĭ) blade, No. 12, is used for opening sinus tracts and fistulae. The No. 15 is used for delicate dissection. There is a long handle that also uses the 10 series blades. It is used for cutting deep structures such as in the pelvis. There is a large handle that uses a larger (20 series) blade.

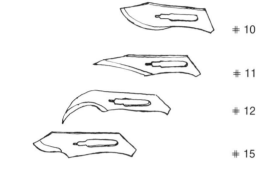

\# 10

\# 11

\# 12

\# 15

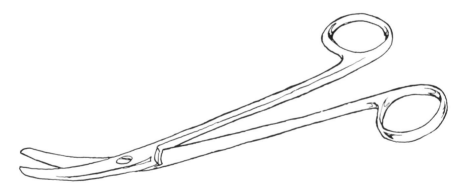

Fig. 4.4   This is a *dissecting scissors,* known by the eponym Metzenbaum. It comes in all sizes from "baby Metz" to "long Metz."

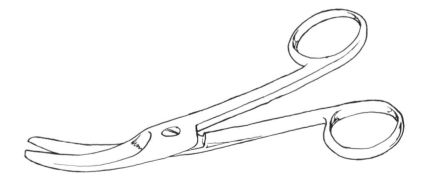

Fig. 4.5   The *heavy scissors* is known as a Mayo. It has curved or straight blunt-tipped blades and is used for cutting heavy structures and sutures.

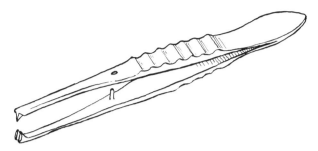

Fig. 4.6   This *heavy-toothed forceps* is known as a rat-tooth forceps. It is used when a firm grasp is more important than gentle tissue handling. It is most commonly used to hold fascia for abdominal wound closure.

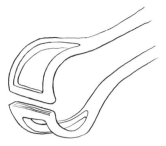

Fig. 4.10   *Babcock clamps* encircle tubular structures and gently hold soft viscera. The ratchet should be tightened only enough to hold the tissue. These are ringed instruments, and only a close-up view of the grasping end is shown.

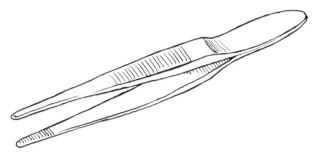

Fig. 4.7   The *plain forceps* has little holding power. It is useful for packing a wound or a cavity.

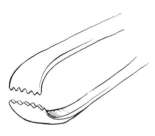

Fig. 4.11   *Allis clamps* have teeth and are somewhat more traumatic than the Babcock.

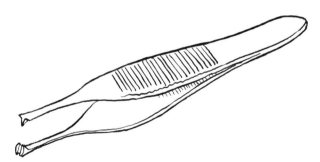

Fig. 4.8   This *small-toothed forceps* is usually referred to as an Adson forceps. It is used for more delicate work where firm fixation is necessary, as in minor surgery. There is a variation with longitudinal rows of smaller teeth, which distribute the force and are less traumatic.

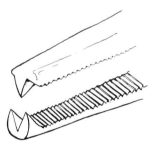

Fig. 4.12   The *Kocher clamp* is a crushing instrument. It is used to hold structures that will be removed.

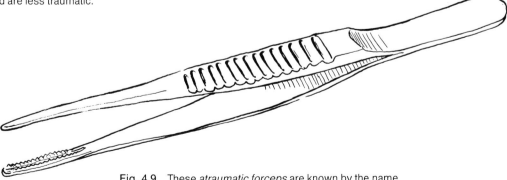

Fig. 4.9   These *atraumatic forceps* are known by the name DeBakey. The tapered flexible blades and rows of small teeth cause minimal injury. They were designed as vascular forceps but are widely used for other tissues.

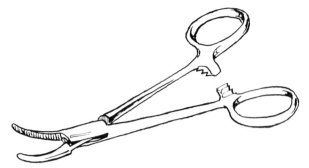

There is a large group of specialized clamps used in vascular surgery. There are also atraumatic gastrointestinal clamps, which will be discussed with the gastrointestinal surgical procedures.

Clamps should be closed one notch before they are returned to the instrument nurse so that they don't fall open and make passing awkward (Fig. 4.12–4.15).

Fig. 4.13 *Mosquito clamps* are used to clamp fine vessels and structures.

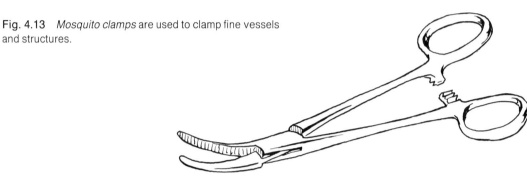

Fig. 4.14 The *hemostat* may be straight or curved and may have teeth covering part or all of the blade. Kelly clamps have teeth only on the distal half of the blades; Crile clamps have teeth all the way up to the blade. Hemostats are used (as the name implies) for securing blood vessels and also for general grasping purposes.

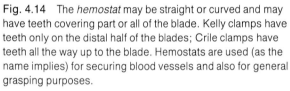
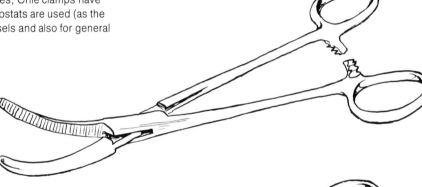

Fig. 4.15 *Large clamps* have a long blade and a blunt tip. Some surgeons use clamps for blunt dissection, but this should be kept to a minimum. Peans and Carmalts are large clamps that have different kinds of teeth.

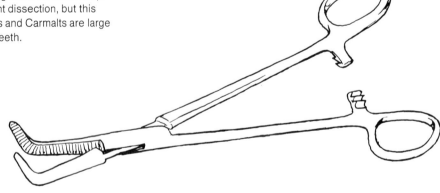

Fig. 4.16 The *right-angle clamp* comes in various sizes with blunt or narrow tips. Its purpose is to get around tubular structures. It is frequently used to pass ligatures. The *tonsil* is a long clamp similar in configuration to a long right-angle clamp but with gently curving blades. It, too, is used as a ligature passer in addition to its primary purpose of clamping deep structures.

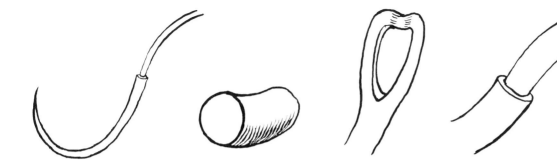

Fig. 4.17 The *taper needle* has a round profile and tapered point, as the name implies. Needles may be straight or curved. The curved needle may have a small or a large arc ($\frac{1}{4}$–$\frac{5}{8}$ circle) and comes in a variety of sizes. Needles with a larger arc are used in confined spaces. The ideal length-to-diameter ratio for maximal strength and minimal trauma is 8:1. The taper needle is used for soft, delicate tissue.

Fig. 4.18 Most sutures available now are swaged onto the needle. Rarely is the older procedure of threading suture material through an eyed needle necessary. The swaged arrangement may be referred to as an atraumatic suture because it is not necessary to pull a double strand of suture material through tissue.

Fig. 4.19 The *cutting needle* is used for tough tissue such as skin. The profile of a curved cutting needle is shown. A reverse cutting needle has the flat side on the inside of the curve. Hand-held, straight cutting needles are discussed with skin suture technique.

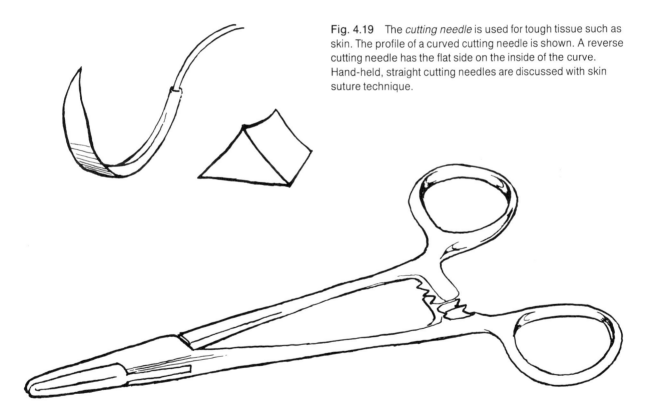

Fig. 4.20 *Needle-holders* are available in many lengths and with gripping surfaces suitable for delicate or heavy work. Needle-holders with angled tips are good for deep, awkward suturing. Some needle-holders have beveled joints to prevent the suture from catching during instrument ties. Some needle shafts are ribbed to mesh with the gripping surface of the needle-holder and prevent rotation.

There are several specialized needle-holders, such as the spring-and-latch microsurgical instrument (Castroviejo) and the plastic ratchetless surgical instrument that incorporates scissor blades behind the grasping surface (Gillies).

Fig. 4.21   *Skin hooks* are self-explanatory and are used for delicate work. (This drawing is enlarged.)

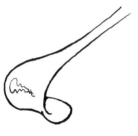

Fig. 4.22   *Vein retractors* are small and smooth bladed. They retract vessels and other cordlike structures.

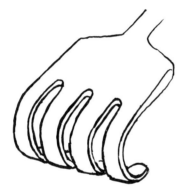

Fig. 4.23   The *rake retractors* have a variable number of teeth and have sharp or dull points. Sharp rakes are more traumatic but hold better; blunt rakes are preferred whenever possible. Rakes are usually used in pairs for superficial work.

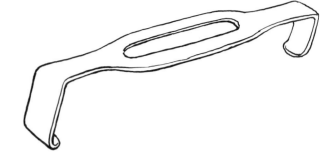

Fig. 4.24   The *Army-Navy retractor* has one long and one short blade.

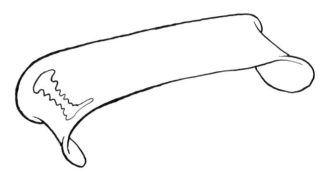

Fig. 4.25   The small flat-bladed retractors are best called by their eponyms. The *Roux* is shown here; the *Halsted* is similar but without the flare at the edges.

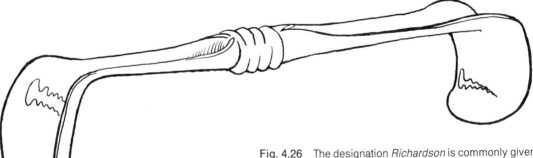

Fig. 4.26   The designation *Richardson* is commonly given both to this double-ended retractor and to its single-ended cousin. It is used primarily for elevating the abdominal wall at the start of a laparotomy.

There are variants such as the *body wall retractor*, which has a broader blade.

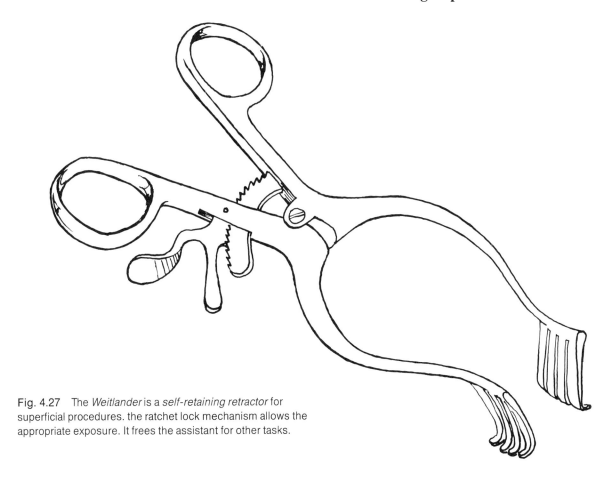

Fig. 4.27   The *Weitlander* is a *self-retaining retractor* for superficial procedures. the ratchet lock mechanism allows the appropriate exposure. It frees the assistant for other tasks.

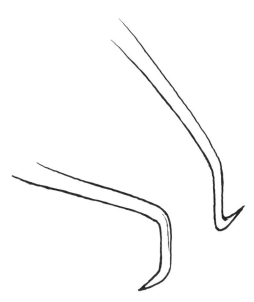

Fig. 4.28   The *Gelpie* is a variant of the self-retaining retractor without the tines of the Weitlander. It doesn't distribute the tension as evenly as the Weitlander, but there is less metal at the business end to interfere with dissection.

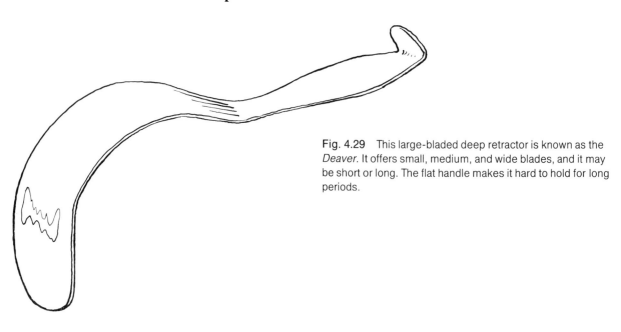

Fig. 4.29   This large-bladed deep retractor is known as the *Deaver*. It offers small, medium, and wide blades, and it may be short or long. The flat handle makes it hard to hold for long periods.

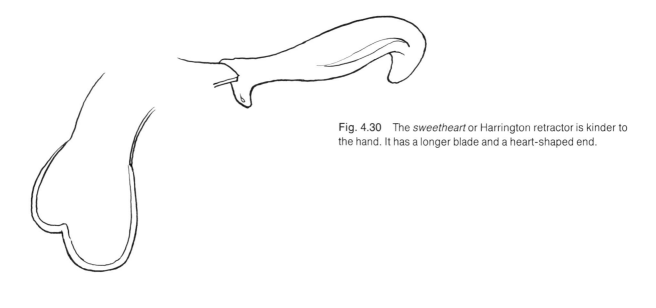

Fig. 4.30   The *sweetheart* or Harrington retractor is kinder to the hand. It has a longer blade and a heart-shaped end.

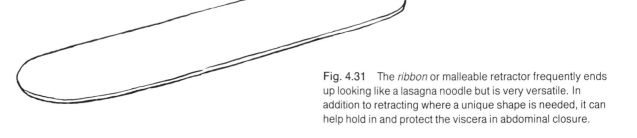

Fig. 4.31   The *ribbon* or malleable retractor frequently ends up looking like a lasagna noodle but is very versatile. In addition to retracting where a unique shape is needed, it can help hold in and protect the viscera in abdominal closure.

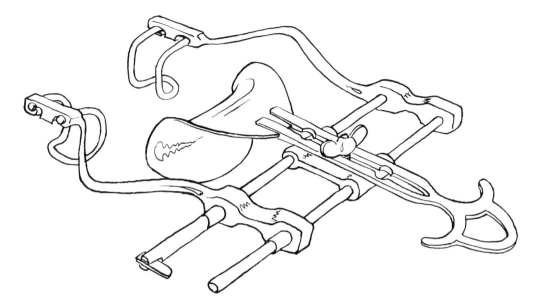

Fig. 4.32 The *Balfour* is a *self-retaining abdominal wall retractor*. There are deep and shallow abdominal wall blades and bladder blades. The abdominal wound edges should be protected with moist pads before the blades are inserted and opened. When opening this type of retractor, one should keep a hand over each blade to avoid trapping viscera between the blade and the abdominal wall. This retractor comes in a regular and a large size.

To prevent abdominal wall tissue injury, care should be taken to use only as much force on a retractor as necessary! Also remember that the greater the exposure and the longer the procedure, the more fluid loss and tissue desiccation you will have. Keep moist pads over everything you are not working on (Fig. 4.20–4.32).

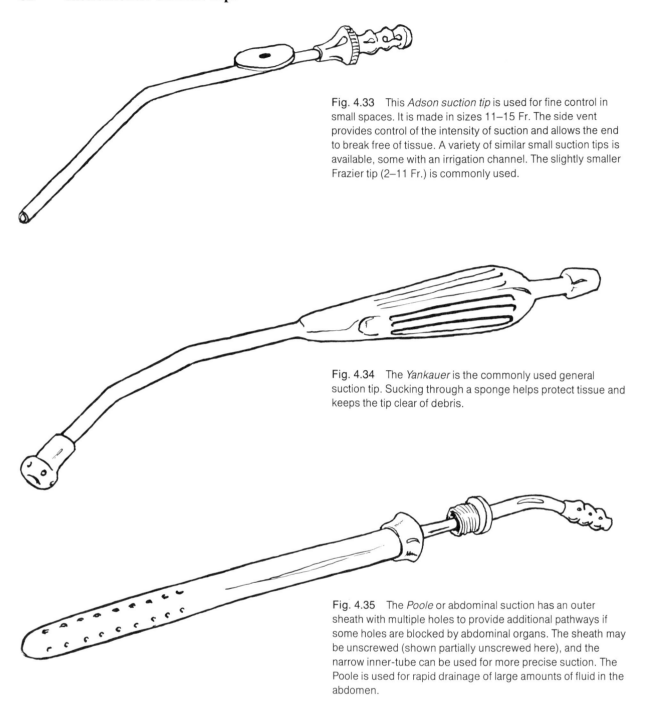

Fig. 4.33   This *Adson suction tip* is used for fine control in small spaces. It is made in sizes 11–15 Fr. The side vent provides control of the intensity of suction and allows the end to break free of tissue. A variety of similar small suction tips is available, some with an irrigation channel. The slightly smaller Frazier tip (2–11 Fr.) is commonly used.

Fig. 4.34   The *Yankauer* is the commonly used general suction tip. Sucking through a sponge helps protect tissue and keeps the tip clear of debris.

Fig. 4.35   The *Poole* or abdominal suction has an outer sheath with multiple holes to provide additional pathways if some holes are blocked by abdominal organs. The sheath may be unscrewed (shown partially unscrewed here), and the narrow inner-tube can be used for more precise suction. The Poole is used for rapid drainage of large amounts of fluid in the abdomen.

Rapid evacuation of large amounts of blood is sometimes necessary. A ruptured spleen or aneurysm may require multiple suckers and lap pads to gain exposure and control.

What suction tips are not is perhaps more important than what they are. A suction tip is not a toy for a bored medical student to use to beat on tissue. Suctioning is not a substitute for hemostasis in obtaining a field clear of blood in which to operate. Suction tips are not retractors or dissectors and should never be used as such (Fig. 4.33–4.35).

Chapter 5

Basic Surgical Maneuvers

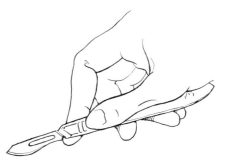

"Chyrurgerie: The quicke motion of an intrepide hand joyned with experience."

Definition quoted by AMBROISE PARÉ, 1582

This section deals with the use of the basic surgical tools and techniques, considered in the following order: scalpel, scissors, forceps, clamp, ligature, needle-holder, suture, hemostatic maneuvers, and retraction. The discussions stress effective use of hands and body position. The specialized function of each instrument is emphasized.

Surgical dissection is a complex art that cannot be learned simply by studying individual skills. Examples of how these skills are coordinated and applied are found in later chapters.

There is a wide range of tissue composition and consequently a variable response to the maneuvers of dissection. In addition, the nature of any tissue may change with disease. References are made to tissue characteristics both in this and in later chapters. The technique must be suited to the tissue.

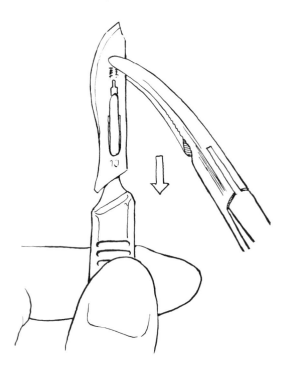

Fig. 5.1   The blade is usually placed on the handle by the scrub nurse unless the surgeon is doing a minor case alone. The body of the blade is held at an acute angle in the jaws of a clamp. The scalpel handle is positioned with the grooved key facing upward. The narrowed portion of the blade opening is gently seated in the grooves, and the blade is slid into place toward the operator.

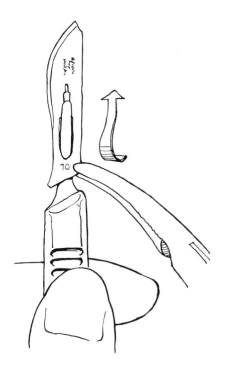

Fig. 5.2   The blade should be changed at the first sign of dullness. The heel of the blade is lifted with the tip of a clamp, and the blade is slipped off away from the operator. The blade must not be pointed toward anyone else during this maneuver.

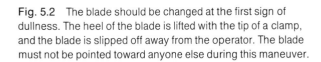

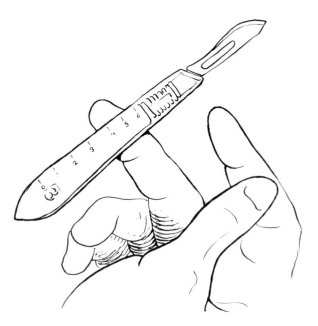

Fig. 5.3   Become familiar with the balance and feel of your instruments. This allows you to position your hand naturally and comfortably. The instrument then becomes a graceful extension of your hand rather than an awkward appliance. A gentle grip affords the best feel of the tissues to which the instrument is applied.

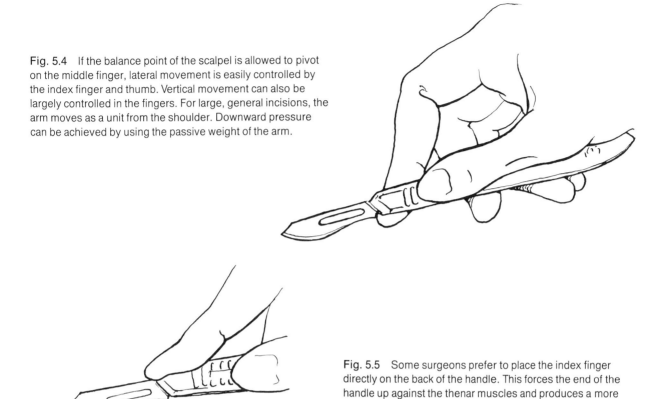

Fig. 5.4 If the balance point of the scalpel is allowed to pivot on the middle finger, lateral movement is easily controlled by the index finger and thumb. Vertical movement can also be largely controlled in the fingers. For large, general incisions, the arm moves as a unit from the shoulder. Downward pressure can be achieved by using the passive weight of the arm.

Fig. 5.5 Some surgeons prefer to place the index finger directly on the back of the handle. This forces the end of the handle up against the thenar muscles and produces a more rigid grip. Lateral and vertical movement is then more dependent on wrist movement. The novice should try each grip and decide which feels more comfortable.

Fig. 5.6 Fine knife dissection is controlled by finger movement. The scalpel is held like a pencil and movement occurs only distal to the metacarpophalangeal (MP) joints. The heel of the hand is firmly seated on adjacent tissue for stability. Dissection should always start in healthy tissue so that relationships remain clear as the pathology is approached.

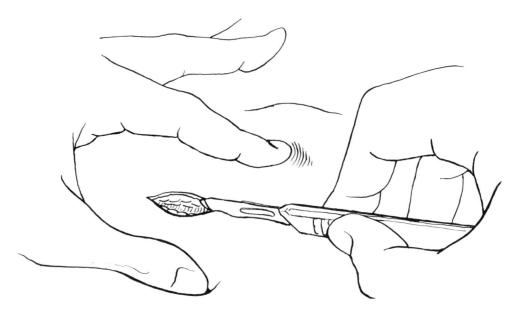

Fig. 5.7   The convex blades cut best with the curve of the belly. The incision is made with a single, smooth, sweeping motion originating at the surgeon's shoulder. Constant pressure results in a uniform depth for each stroke.

Just as in a sport, preparation is as important as the execution of a move. Position your body so that the incision can be completed comfortably. The right-handed surgeon is most comfortable with an incision from left to right and toward himself. The surgeon would therefore stand slightly away from the table and facing the patient's flank for a subcostal incision. For a midline incision he would turn his body perpendicular to the table with his right hip adjacent to the patient's right hip.

Steadily increasing traction by surgeon and assistant opens up the developing incision.

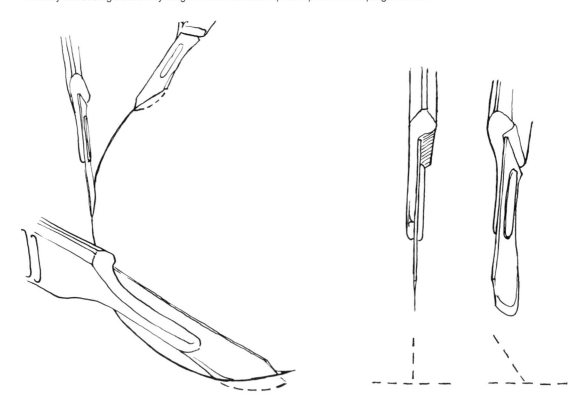

Fig. 5.8   Change in direction – for example, going around the umbilicus with a midline incision – is accomplished by turning body and arm while keeping the knife blade perpendicular to skin. Elevating the handle allows the cut to be made by a shorter arc of the blade (nearer the tip) and facilitates turning a curve.

Fig. 5.9   The blade should be kept perpendicular to the structure being cut. A beveled skin edge results in uneven closure and may lead to necrosis at the beveled edge. The first cut should go through skin. A new blade is used for the rest of the incision. Compared with blunt means of dissecting tissue planes – finger, gauze, clamp – the knife is the least traumatic.

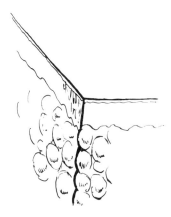

Fig. 5.10 A clean, vertical incision leaves sharply transected blood vessels, which can contract effectively.

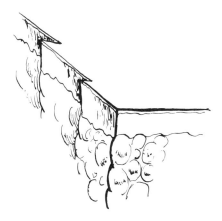

Fig. 5.11 A jagged incision results from choppy, hesitating movements by the surgeon. When the surgeon hesitates, the assistant may change traction and accentuate the effect. The knife should not be lifted while the initial skin incision is being made.

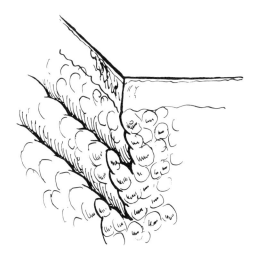

Fig. 5.12 If the assistant pulls unevenly as the incision is deepened, each new sweep of the knife falls in a different line. A terraced effect with excessive devitalized fat results.

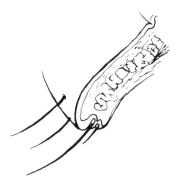

Fig. 5.13 Skin thickness varies significantly in different parts of the body. The pressure on the knife must be consistent with the nature of the tissue. Skin of the eyelid and of some elderly patients is thin and delicate.

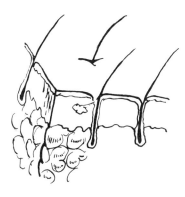

Fig. 5.14 Skin over most of the extremities, abdomen, chest, and face is a few millimeters thick.

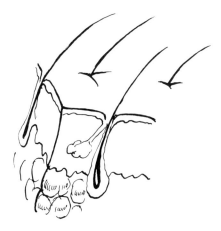

Fig. 5.15 The skin of the scalp and back is the thickest of the body, sometimes measuring several millimeters. This alters the surgical approach to various skin and subcutaneous lesions.

Fig. 5.16 This and the following two illustrations demonstrate the 180° arc between full pronation and full supination. This movement is basic in the use of all ringed instruments. Rotation in the axis of the forearm provides a complete range of positions for the tip of the scissors. The body should be turned freely to maintain this axial relationship between scissors and forearm. The cut is most natural and therefore most controlled when the surgeon cuts away from himself and from right to left (the opposite of knife dissection).

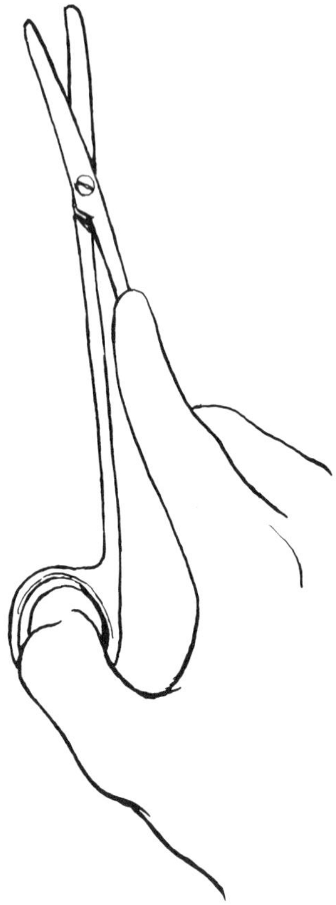

Fig. 5.17 When the situation favors a vertical position for the scissors, the points may face right or left, extending the range of point positions to 360°.

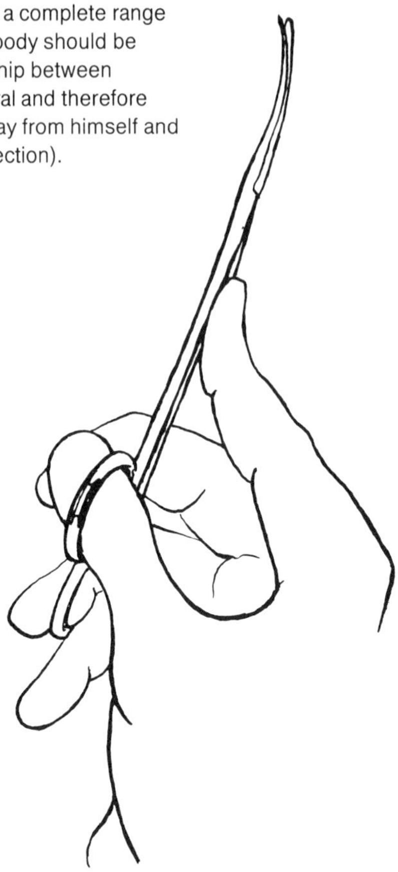

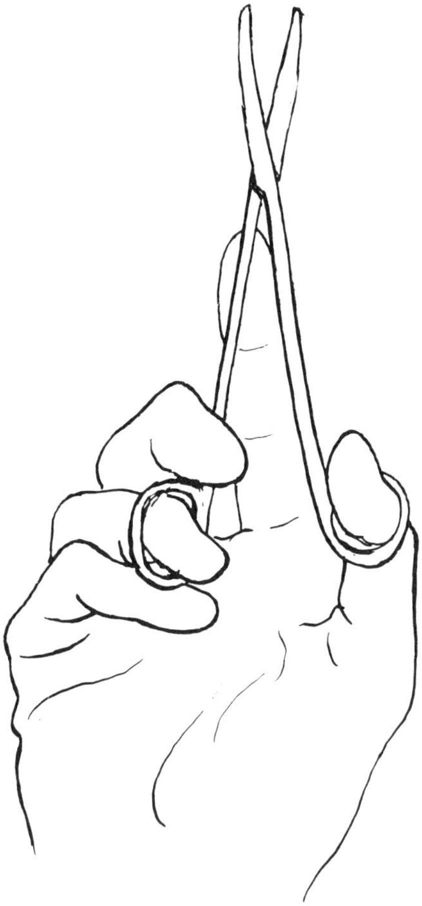

Fig. 5.18 Supination puts slightly more strain on the fine control of the hand.

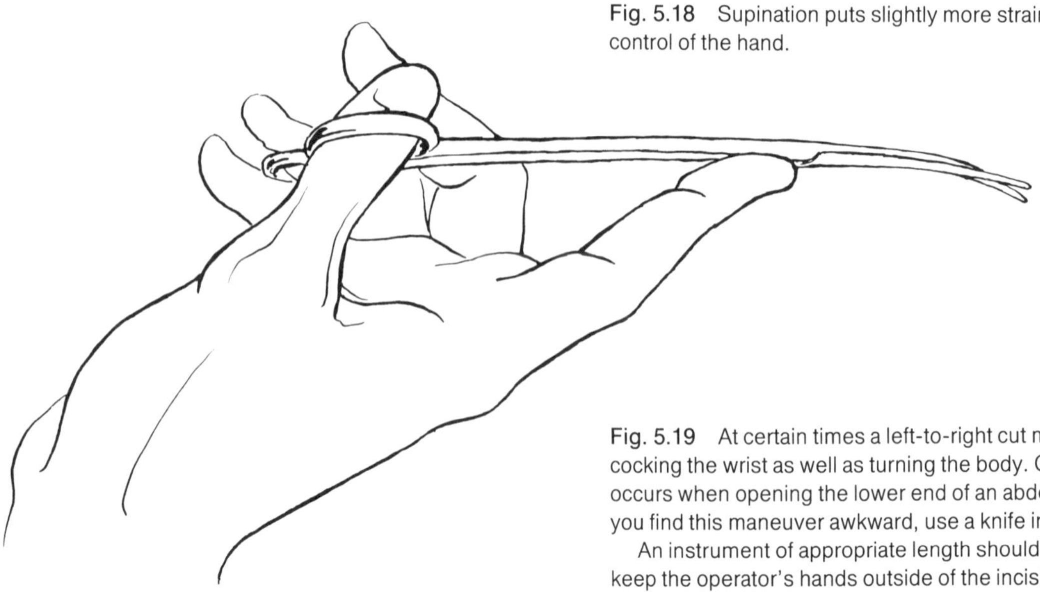

Fig. 5.19 At certain times a left-to-right cut may necessitate cocking the wrist as well as turning the body. One such time occurs when opening the lower end of an abdominal incision. If you find this maneuver awkward, use a knife instead.

An instrument of appropriate length should be chosen to keep the operator's hands outside of the incision.

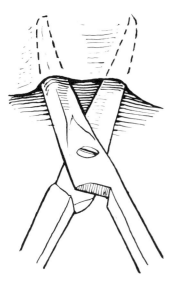

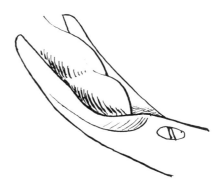

Fig. 5.22   The heavy Mayo scissors is used for cutting tough structures and for bulk debridement. Some soft tissues (such as necrotic muscle) that cannot be grasped directly may be excised by pressing down with the heel of the scissors.

Fig. 5.20   The Metzenbaum scissors is used for general dissection. Pressure is applied to the rings in such a way that the cutting edges are kept firmly apposed. Blunt dissection should only be used to define a natural tissue plane. A single gentle spread should open just enough space for the subsequent cut. Forceful stretching will tear adjacent vessels and structures.

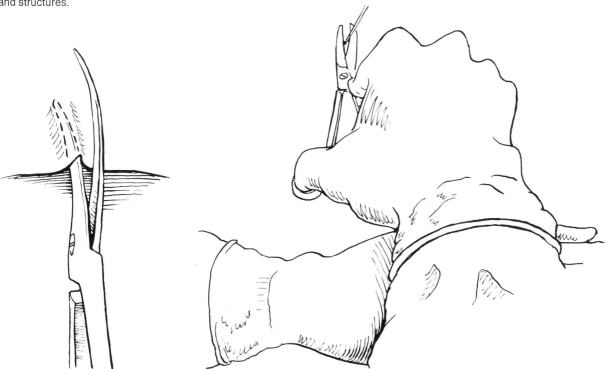

Fig. 5.21   The scissors is withdrawn and turned 90°; then the lower blade is reinserted. The tip should go no further than the previous dissection. The structure should be held tense to ensure a clean cut. The cut is completed with a single smooth motion.

Fig. 5.23   Heavy blunt-tipped scissors are also used to cut sutures. The assistant should ask the surgeon how long to cut a particular suture if he is uncertain. The suture should be held so that it does not obscure the assistant's view of the knot. Accurate placement of the scissors tip under direct vision is facilitated by steadying the forearm on the other hand. The scissors tip should be held close by as the knot is completed and should not be pulled away until it is clear that the suture is cleanly cut.

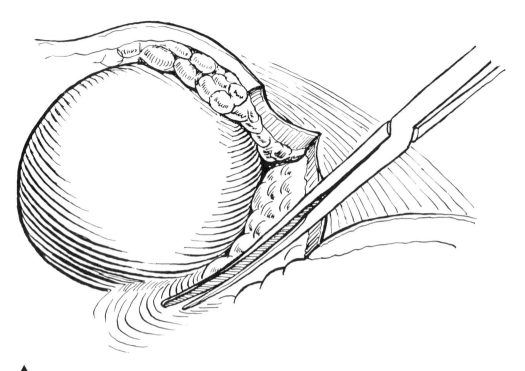

▲
Fig. 5.24   Attempting to dissect flexible structures without proper fixation and retraction can be like trying to excise a marble from a block of gelatin. The more you push, the more the walls close in on you. The points of the scissors are buried and cutting is almost impossible.

Fig. 5.25   The basic principle of exposure is two-point traction. In many cases one of the two points is a relatively fixed feature of the anatomy. An example is the adhesions between gallbladder and liver. The gallbladder is put on stretch; the liver bed remains the fixed point. In most cases two points of traction are needed around soft structures, as shown here. The objectives are to demonstrate the anatomy clearly, to expose adjacent structures that may otherwise be injured, to allow dissection and hemostasis under direct vision, and to stretch tissues so they can be cleanly cut.
▼

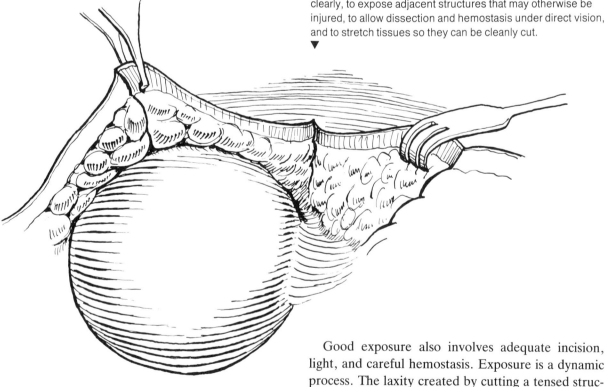

Good exposure also involves adequate incision, light, and careful hemostasis. Exposure is a dynamic process. The laxity created by cutting a tensed structure must be counteracted by applying more traction to maintain a steady state.

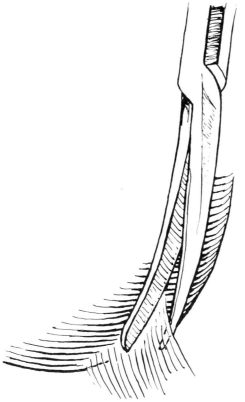

Fig. 5.26   The curve of the scissors should follow the curve of the structure being dissected. A small nick is often needed to enter the proper fascial plane.

Fig. 5.27   To dissect around a curved structure such as a cyst, a small tunnel is created following the natural shape. Dissection proceeds one layer at a time. Each layer is completed before the next is entered so that you don't work yourself into a hole.

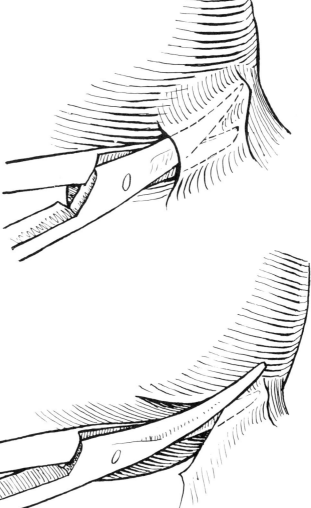

Fig. 5.28   The frenulum created by the blunt dissection is divided.

In the following pages the use of grasping instruments is discussed. There is necessarily some overlap with hemostasis and knot tying. Figures 5.35 through 5.39 describe isolation, clamping, and dividing of a tubular structure.

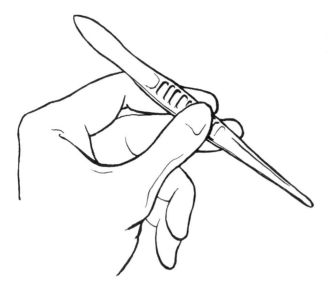

Fig. 5.29 The forceps, like the scalpel, is held with a gentle, balanced grip. If you have to squeeze hard to hold a particular tissue, either you are using the wrong kind of forceps or a clamp would be more appropriate.

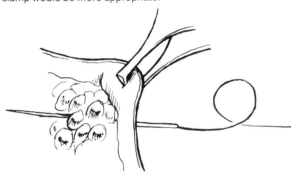

Fig. 5.30 A fine-toothed forceps such as an Adson is used for a moderately dense tissue such as skin. The points concentrate force on a tiny area and give more holding power with less tissue destruction than could be obtained with a blunt forceps.

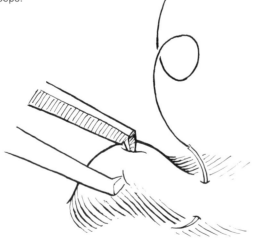

Fig. 5.31 A dense fascia, as exists along the abdominal midline, requires a heavier-toothed forceps. The forceps is placed so that it stabilizes the tissue immediately adjacent to the site where a stitch is to be placed.

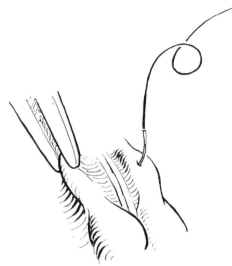

Fig. 5.32 Delicate tissue such as mucosa is gently handled with multiple small teeth as found in the DeBakey tissue forceps. The force is distributed and adequate holding power is maintained.

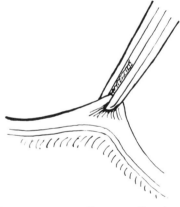

Fig. 5.33 Forceps may grasp the supporting structures of a nerve but never the nerve itself.

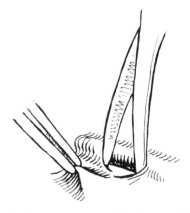

Fig. 5.34 The forceps serves as the principal tool for fine retraction during dissection.

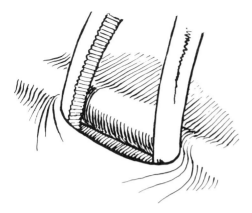

Fig. 5.35 Clamps may be used for dissection in very loose areolar tissue such as retroperitoneum, but in most instances the knife or scissors is more precise and less traumatic.

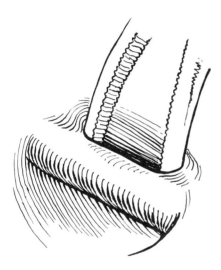

Fig. 5.36 Small spreading movements parallel to the structure will prevent tearing of branches. Some advocate spreading perpendicular to vessels for the same reason. A length is prepared that is long enough to be securely clamped and safely divided.

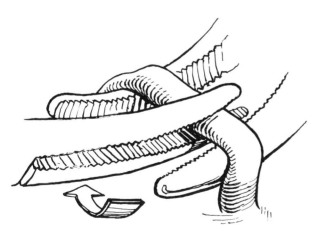

Fig. 5.37 The structure is elevated on an open clamp. A second clamp is placed in position. One jaw of the supporting clamp is lowered.

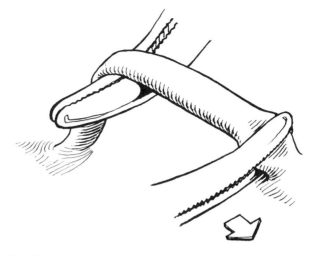

Fig. 5.38 The second clamp can then be moved to the end of the dissected segment and clamped. A small amount of tip is left exposed beyond the structure to facilitate ligation. The opposite end is clamped with the original clamp.

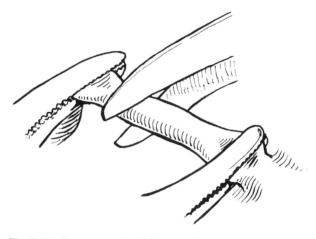

Fig. 5.39 The structure is divided, leaving the longer stump on the business end (proximal to an artery) so that it can be easily found if it escapes. If the structure is not ligated immediately, the ring end of the clamp is placed out of the way toward the periphery of the wound. It can be covered so that sutures do not get snagged on the rings.

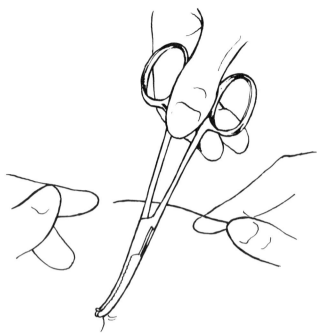

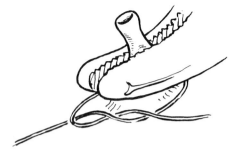

Fig. 5.42   The tips are elevated and exposed without pulling. The first throw is placed just below the clamp; the strands are oriented parallel to the axis of the clamp.

Fig. 5.40   When dealing with multiple clamps, take the most accessible one first and proceed in logical order. The clamp is elevated without pulling on the clamped structure. The ligature is passed behind.

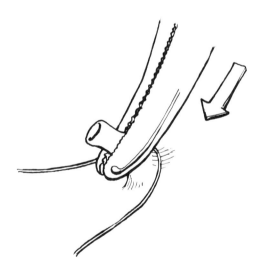

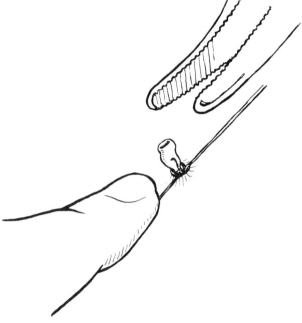

Fig. 5.43   The knot is tightened and tension is maintained as the clamp is slowly released. A few small, quick tugs are most effective for securing each throw without breaking the suture material. There is extra give as the tissue splayed by the clamp is released. Note that the two strands and the knot form a straight line, and no tension is placed on the vessel. If the vessel is large, it may be advisable to flash (open and reclamp) the clamp and place a second tie or suture ligature.

A good assistant should be able to control the release of a clamp with either hand.

Fig. 5.41   The ligature is slid down the heel of the clamp as the clamp is lowered to a horizontal position. If the clamped structure is too deep to trap the strand before tying, the first throw may be made high on the clamp and slid down into position.

Fig. 5.44 When tying a structure in continuity (as opposed to tying a cut structure) or when tying around a deeply placed clamp, a ligature must be passed. The end of the ligature is clamped in the tip of the passing instrument (usually a long clamp like a tonsil). The ligature is stretched like a bow string across the ratchet and held with the thumb. The passer is opened and the free end of the ligature is pulled through. When passing a ligature around a deep clamp tip, the free end of the ligature rather than the passing instrument is passed behind the ring end of the clamp first.

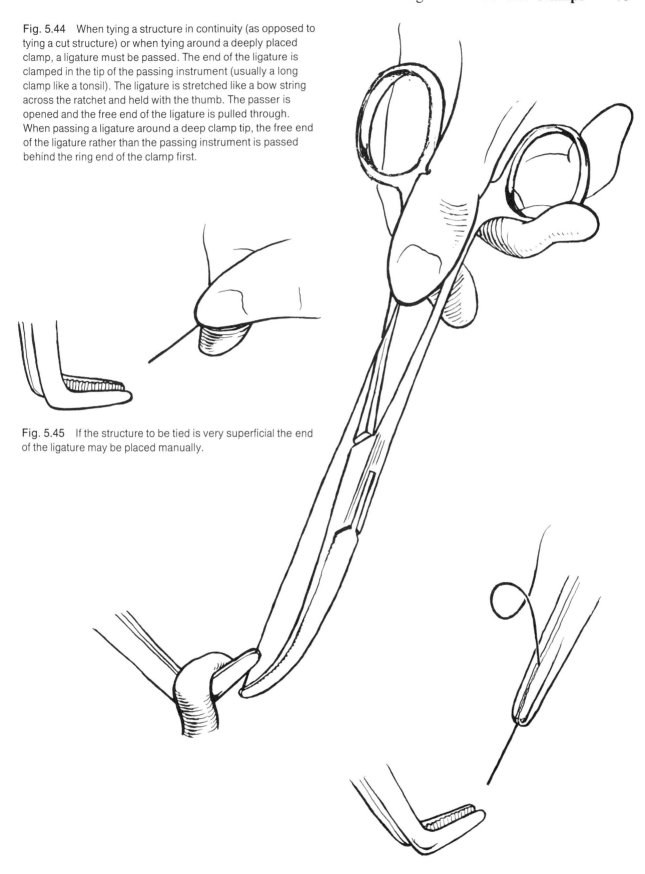

Fig. 5.45 If the structure to be tied is very superficial the end of the ligature may be placed manually.

Fig. 5.46 Using a long forceps eliminates the need to unclamp the passing instrument.

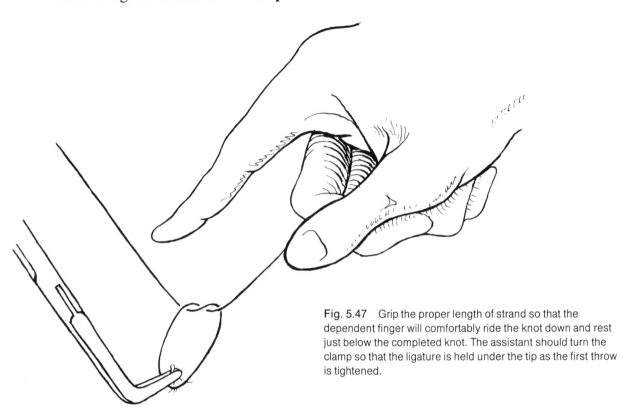

Fig. 5.47 Grip the proper length of strand so that the dependent finger will comfortably ride the knot down and rest just below the completed knot. The assistant should turn the clamp so that the ligature is held under the tip as the first throw is tightened.

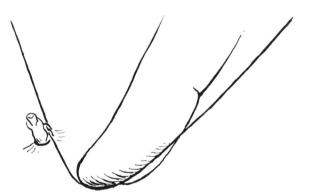

Fig. 5.48 The straight-line relationship is maintained. The dependent finger controls the position of the knot so that the ligated structure is not avulsed. During the execution of a good knot, the structure being tied should not move at all.

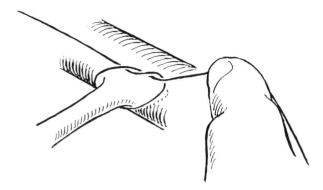

Fig. 5.49   To tie a branch flush with the main vessel, the dependent finger places slight traction toward the parent structure just as the first throw is tightened. This compensates for the tendency of the knot to slide off the sloping shoulder of the junction. If the branch is put under tension, the parent structure can be tented and its lumen can be compromised.

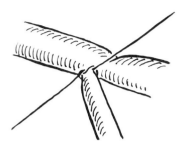

Fig. 5.51   Crossing a strand over the main vessel may lead to injury such as intimal damage and thrombosis in a vein.

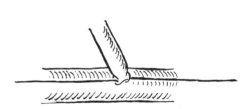

Fig. 5.50   The knot should be completed with the strands parallel to the main vessel.

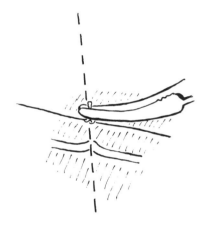

Fig. 5.52   The strands must be kept parallel to an adjacent nerve. Crossing the nerve with a taut strand (dotted line) could cause damage. This situation is commonly encountered with the recurrent laryngeal nerve during thyroidectomy.

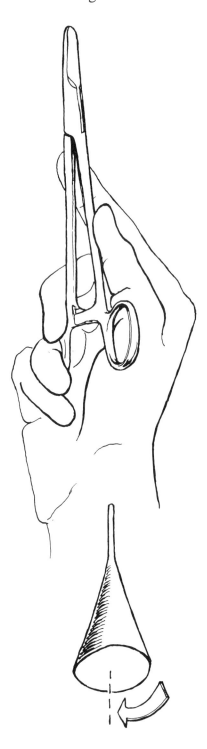

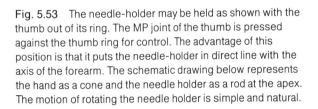

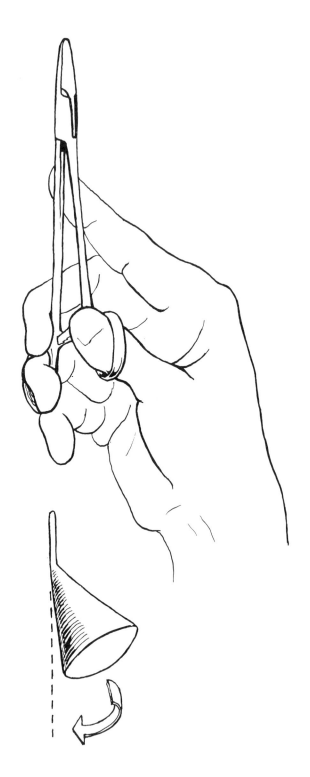

Fig. 5.53   The needle-holder may be held as shown with the thumb out of its ring. The MP joint of the thumb is pressed against the thumb ring for control. The advantage of this position is that it puts the needle-holder in direct line with the axis of the forearm. The schematic drawing below represents the hand as a cone and the needle holder as a rod at the apex. The motion of rotating the needle holder is simple and natural.

Fig. 5.54   Traditionally the thumb is kept in the ring. The schematic below shows that the rotation of the needle-holder on its axis requires a more complex movement of hand, wrist, and forearm. The individual surgeon must choose the method that works best for him.

Fig. 5.55 The needle should enter a structure at right angles to its surface. In the case of skin, this involves pushing firmly downward until dermis is penetrated, then turning.

In special circumstances the needle may be angulated in the jaws for a better entry position. For general use the needle is grasped closer to the suture than to the point. For dense tissue and vascular suturing, the needle is held closer to its middle.

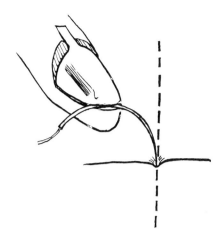

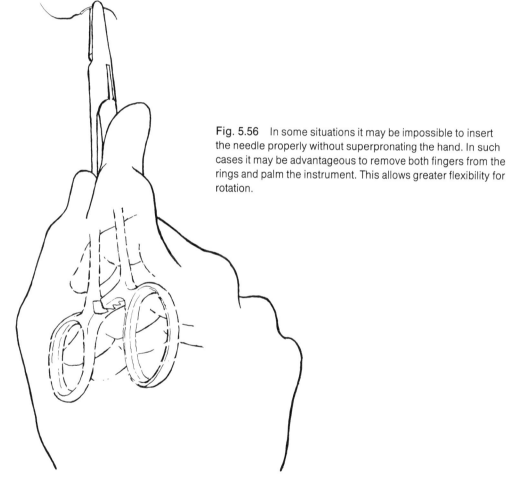

Fig. 5.56 In some situations it may be impossible to insert the needle properly without superpronating the hand. In such cases it may be advantageous to remove both fingers from the rings and palm the instrument. This allows greater flexibility for rotation.

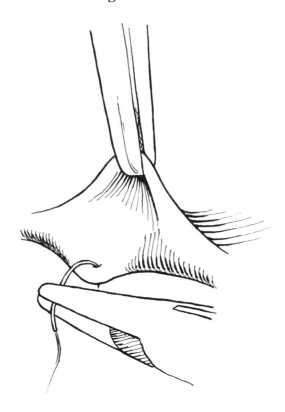

Fig. 5.57   This figure shows a situation in which freehand use of the needle holder is beneficial. The first layer of the Shouldice hernia repair uses the reflected edge of the transversalis fascia, which lies posterior to the transversus muscle. To get a solid bite of this tissue, the initial direction of the needle point must be almost anterior. The needle tip should be placed accurately the first time to avoid multiple puncture wounds. The needle should be passed smoothly in an arc dictated by its curve. The passage is complete when the needle-holder is stopped by the tissue.

   The forceps stabilizing the adjacent tissue is providing countertraction, which allows easy passage. The traction then keeps the needle in position and provides exposure for easy withdrawal. The forceps should not change position until the needle is withdrawn.

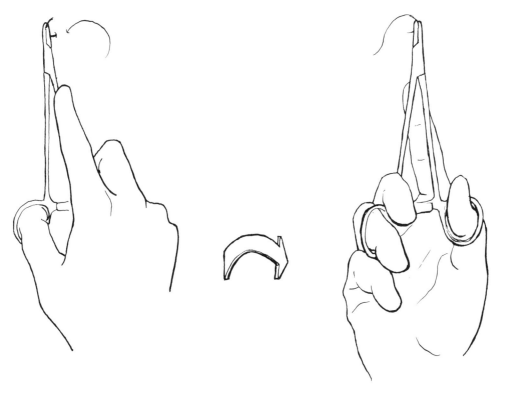

Fig. 5.58   To withdraw a curved needle, the hand starts in the pronated position. The needle is removed in a small arc that follows its curve. In the process the hand turns 180° to supination. The movement is natural and minimal, involving only the forearm.

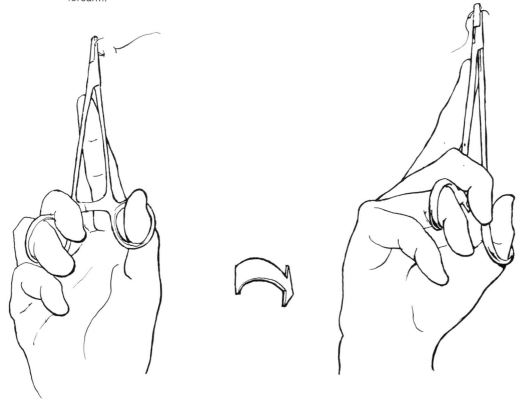

Fig. 5.59   If the needle is initially grasped with the hand supinated, withdrawal requires complex movement. The wrist, forearm, elbow, brachium, and shoulder must all change position, resulting in an awkward hypersupination.

Several basic suture patterns are presented in Figs. 5.60–5.73, with elaboration on skin suture technique. Stitches used for abdominal closure and retention sutures are discussed in the chapter on laparotomy.

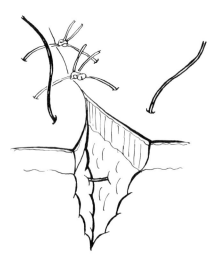

Fig. 5.60 The *simple suture* should have a square profile to avoid inverting skin edges. This is accomplished as shown in Figs. 5.64–5.68. A good general rule for placement is that the width of each stitch equals the distance between sutures. The width varies with the thickness of the skin, the location, and the purpose of the suture.

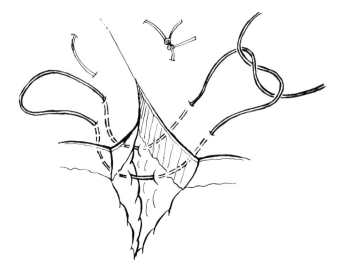

Fig. 5.62 The *horizontal mattress* is an everting stitch that is more commonly used in fascia than in skin.

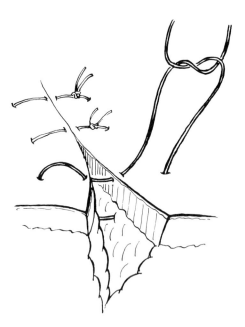

Fig. 5.61 The *vertical mattress* is used when precise edge approximation is important and cannot be achieved with a simple suture. This is the most common skin closure pattern. It consists of two tiny epidermal-thickness bites of the edges, added to the simple suture. Gentle, loose approximation allows for the edema that inevitably follows wounding.

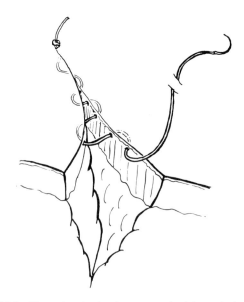

Fig. 5.63 The *subcuticular closure* may be interrupted or continuous. It may be done with absorbable or nonabsorbable material. In the former case the end knot is usually buried. The technique is discussed in more detail in the section on minor surgery.

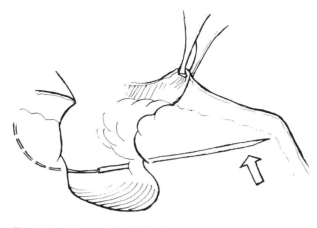

Fig. 5.66 The needle point is elevated, and the subcutaneous tissue is dragged back toward the exit site, causing it to bunch up.

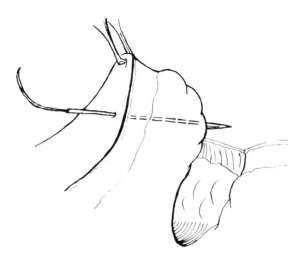

Fig. 5.64 A straight needle is most efficient for skin suture. The flap toward the surgeon or to his right is gently rolled back with a toothed forceps. This allows the needle to pass away from the surgeon and parallel to the cut edge of the wound (perpendicular to the skin surface).

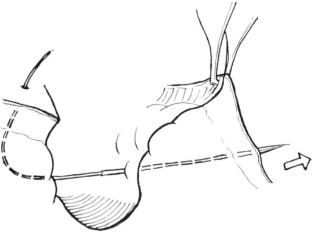

Fig. 5.67 The needle is advanced through the skin. The exit point should be the same distance from the edge as the entry point. If a mattress suture is required, the forceps is not released. The needle is passed back through the skin edge adjacent to the forceps where stability is greatest. A similar bite on the opposite side enters at the dermal-epidermal junction and exits about 1 mm from the edge.

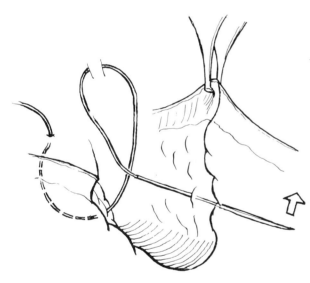

Fig. 5.65 The far edge is elevated, and the needle penetrates the fat at the same depth as on the opposite side. The needle is advanced parallel to the skin surface to a distance beyond the intended exit site.

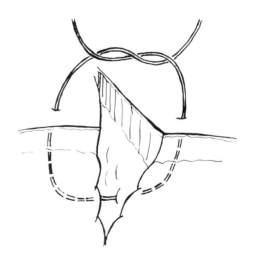

Fig. 5.68 The result is a square-shaped suture that encloses an equal area of dermis on both sides and prevents the edges from inverting. If two people are closing skin, one starts in the center of the incision and the other at the end, and both work in the same direction. They thus remain an equal distance apart and do not get in each other's way.

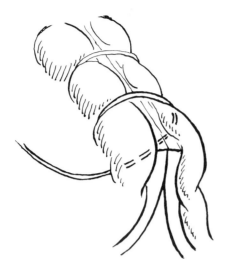

Fig. 5.69   The simple over and over *continuous suture* is the one most often used on bowel. The continuous suture is quicker than the interrupted suture and may distribute tension more evenly. Care must be exercised not to pull too tightly, however, or a rigid purse string results, which can compromise the lumen at an anastomosis. Another disadvantage of continuous suture is that a single break compromises the entire suture line. The needle should be released and the suture should be periodically untwisted when doing a long continuous row. The surgeon sets the tension for each stitch of a continuous suture, and the assistant holds the strand at that tension while the next stitch is placed.

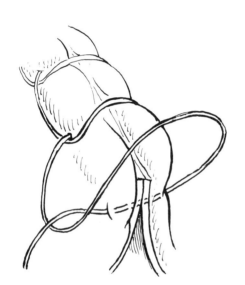

Fig. 5.70   A *continuous locking suture* is created by passing the needle through the loop of the previous stitch. The purpose is to prevent slippage and to aid hemostasis in a cut edge. The assistant flips the loop over so that the surgeon automatically withdraws the needle through it.

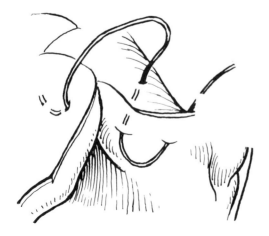

Fig. 5.71   The *Connell* stitch is a continuous inverting suture commonly used for the first layer (anterior wall portion) of a bowel anastomosis. The technique is discussed with small-bowel resection.

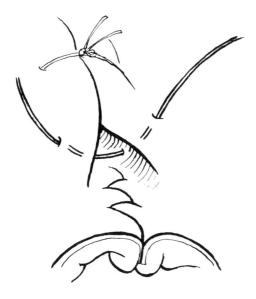

Fig. 5.72   The *Lembert* stitch incorporates the seromuscular
layer and submucosa (the strong collagen-containing layer). It
may be interrupted or continuous and is used for the outer
layer of anastomoses. A stitch should include both sides in one
bite only when the tissue is flexible and well apposed. If the
first side is stressed by an attempt to pass through both sides,
you are sacrificing gentleness and accuracy, and the needle
will probably retract from the second side, negating any time
saving. Never hesitate to take two bites.

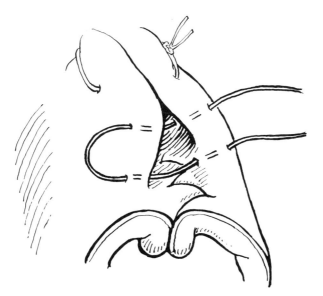

Fig. 5.73   The *Halsted* stitch is an interrupted seromuscular
horizontal mattress. A continuous horizontal mattress is called
a *Cushing* stitch.

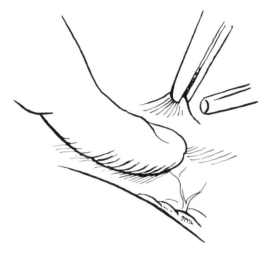

Fig. 5.74   Pressure on a gauze sponge or pad is the first temporizing measure while an incision is being made. Many minor bleeders (especially at the skin edge) will have stopped by the time they are examined. Fingertip pressure with glove rubber directly on the bleeder has the advantage of not pulling off formed clot. The finger is not removed until the means are at hand to deal with the bleeder, i.e., suction, retraction, hemostat, electrocoagulation, clip, or ligature. There is no advantage in repeatedly releasing pressure on a bleeding point just to see if it is still bleeding. A folded gauze sponge on a ring clamp is useful to apply pressure in a deep location.

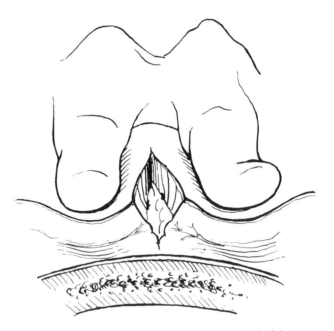

Fig. 5.75   In certain instances, such as in a scalp incision, finger pressure against a hard underlying structure can temporarily control exuberant small bleeders.

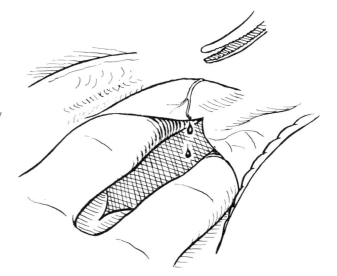

Fig. 5.76 Bleeders in a flat structure such as peritoneum or rectus muscle may sometimes be controlled and visualized by tenting up the structure on two fingers. Relax tension to pinpoint the bleeder when you are ready to clamp.

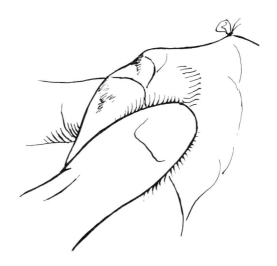

Fig. 5.77 By pinching either side of a mesentery, bleeders in the edge can be controlled. This is a useful maneuver if a large mesenteric vessel escapes and retracts. The same principle is applied in the Pringle maneuver, in which the hepatoduodenal ligament is pinched to decrease massive hepatic bleeding.

The various topical cellulose and collagen hemostatic agents are used to control bleeding from a raw vascular surface such as liver or spleen.

Hemostatic metal clips are used for small deep bleeders. Some operators use clips where multiple small vessels must be divided, such as dividing the short gastric vessels for splenectomy. There are several disadvantages to using clips, however. They are easily dislodged, especially when further manipula-tion of the tissue is necessary. They can get in the way – for example, if placed near the common duct prior to choledochotomy. In that same situation they may interfere with visualization of the cholangiogram. The fact that metal clips are radiopaque is beneficial when they are used to mark the margins of a tumor for later radiotherapy. If used for speed in dividing multiple vessels, clips are best applied only on the side coming out.

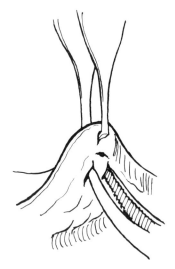

Fig. 5.78   Persistent subcutaneous bleeders (which run in a subdermal plexus) are clamped by fixing the bleeder between the clamp tips and the firm dermis above.

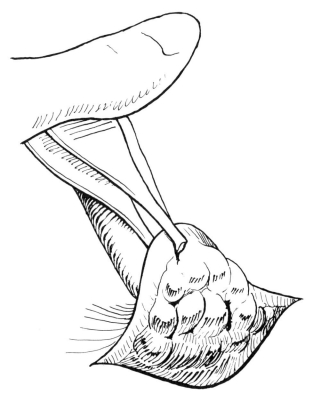

Fig. 5.79   The sides of a deep wound should be rechecked for bleeding at the end of a procedure by eversion with fingertip pressure. This is especially important where there is soft fatty tissue folding in upon itself, as in a breast biopsy.

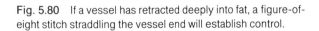

Fig. 5.80   If a vessel has retracted deeply into fat, a figure-of-eight stitch straddling the vessel end will establish control.

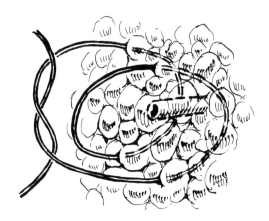

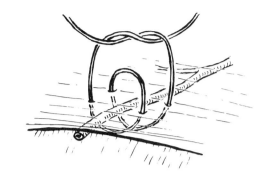

Fig. 5.81 Some bleeding vessels lie in a fascial plane that should not be disturbed by clamping or dissection. An example is the gastroduodenal artery in the bed of a posterior duodenal ulcer. In such cases a figure-of-eight stitch encircling the vessel is appropriate.

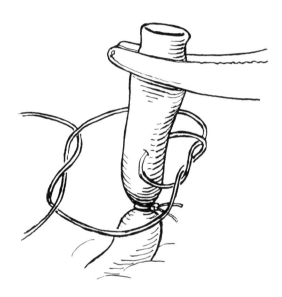

Fig. 5.82 The suture ligature transfixes a large vessel. It is tied on either side and provides security against pulsatile pressure popping off a ligature. It may also be passed around the first side without tying. The vessel is usually tied first, and the suture ligature is then placed distal to the tie. As noted earlier, Halsted pointed out that the security gained by transfixing a vessel permitted the use of finer suture material and avoided the need to forcefully crush the tissues with a larger ligature.

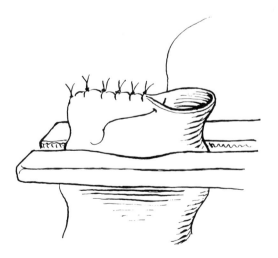

Fig. 5.83 Large vessels are best closed by precise interrupted sutures at the cut end.

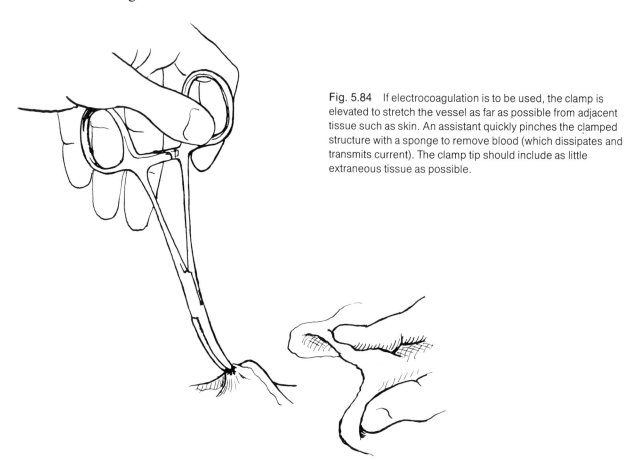

Fig. 5.84   If electrocoagulation is to be used, the clamp is elevated to stretch the vessel as far as possible from adjacent tissue such as skin. An assistant quickly pinches the clamped structure with a sponge to remove blood (which dissipates and transmits current). The clamp tip should include as little extraneous tissue as possible.

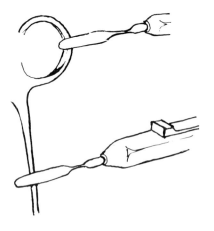

Fig. 5.85   The electrosurgical tip can touch any part of the clamp. The only requirement is that the instrument tip remain clearly visible so that current can be cut off as soon as the effect is achieved. Coagulation is accomplished by the heating resulting from intermittent current. (In the cutting mode the tip delivers a continuous current that superheats and divides local tissue before sufficient heat for coagulation can build up in adjacent tissue.)

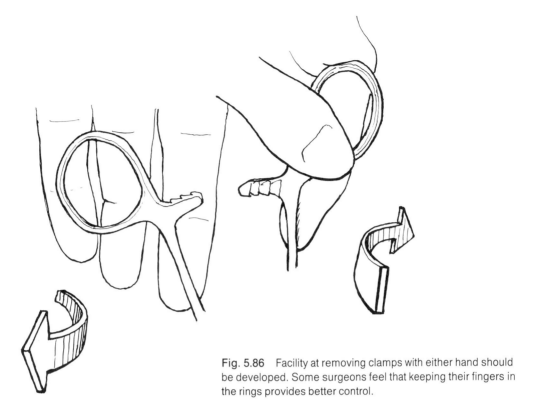

Fig. 5.86   Facility at removing clamps with either hand should be developed. Some surgeons feel that keeping their fingers in the rings provides better control.

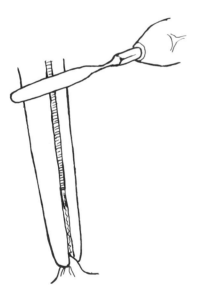

Fig. 5.87   Using a fine-tipped forceps is a quick way of coagulating multiple small bleeders.

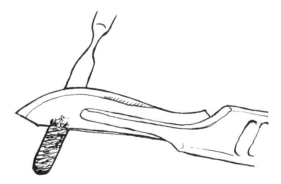

Fig. 5.88   It the coagulation tip is applied directly to bleeding points, the tip will need to be periodically scraped clean. A coagulated structure should not be wiped with a sponge lest the coagulum be dislodged and bleeding be restarted. Dab if necessary.

Electrocoagulation is properly used when it results in less tissue damage than would be caused by a ligature. Attempts to use electrocoagulation on too large a vessel result in an extensive burn and high probability that the vessel will rebleed.

Retraction

There are a few simple principles that apply to the use of retractors. The human hand is by far the best retractor. It is softly padded, gentle, and responsive to the texture of the tissue retracted. When manual retraction is not appropriate, one must choose a retractor of the proper size and shape for the task at hand. Tissues must be insulated by moist pads from the hard metal of the retractor. Retraction must always be gentle to tissue. Excessive, prolonged pressure kills cells, injures small blood vessels, causes temporary or permanent nerve damage, and may rupture the capsule of solid viscera. If excessive traction seems necessary for exposure, the incision is too small.

Hand-held and self-retaining retractors each have advantages and disadvantages. With hand-held retractors the assistant has continuous control and can make precise adjustments. He can also relax tension on tissues at appropriate moments. The great 17th-century samurai Musashi wrote, "Fixedness means a dead hand. Pliability is a living hand." The quality of hand-held retraction is limited by fatigue and by the ability of the assistant to see what he is retracting. Self-retaining retractors maintain a fixed position indefinitely and free the assistants for other tasks. However, they do not allow rapid adjustment or periodic relief of the tissue being retracted. They are also more bulky than hand-held retractors.

Chapter 6

The Surgical Assistant

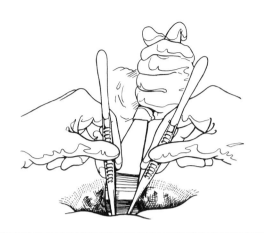

"Those about the patient must present the part to be operated upon as may seem proper and they must hold the rest of body steady, in silence, and listening to the commands of the operator."

HIPPOCRATES (460–380 B.C.)

The best assistant is a good surgeon. The surgeon who is confident of his own mastery of technical principles knows how to provide the services he himself would want. He knows how to get good exposure, how to handle tissues, and how to achieve hemostasis efficiently. Most important, a good surgeon has the patience and maturity to allow his colleague to set the pace and control the direction of the operation without interfering. There are often several solutions to a technical problem, and it is tempting to suggest one's own preferred method to the surgeon when he seems bogged down. The assistant must weigh the benefit of the suggestion against the potential disruption of the surgeon's concentration and rhythm. The better the relationship between surgeon and assistant, the freer the exchange of ideas.

The surgical assistant has a profound impact on the progress of an operation. A good assistant can improve the performance of a less accomplished surgeon and make a good surgeon look like a master. A bad assistant, on the other hand, can make the best surgeon appear awkward. The ideal situation – one good surgeon assisting another – is the exception rather than the rule, especially in centers with training programs.

During medical school and early surgical training, the neophyte is a second or even third assistant. This type of participation could be called primary-level assistance. As the resident gains experience and skill, the quality of his assistance improves and he is given increasing responsibility in increasingly complex cases. When he is capable of advanced assistance, he assumes the position of first assistant. The third category of assisting requires the ability to be more than a skillful first assistant; it involves assisting as an instructor, a responsibility that carries with it many subtle problems.

Primary-Level Assisting

The medical student on his first surgical rotation is often filled with enthusiasm at the prospect of participating in the drama of surgery. This enthusiasm can be easily dispelled if the student is treated as a body attached to the end of a retractor, far out of sight of the operation in progress. The more complex the case, the more minor the student's role must be, but there are ways to prevent the alienation that commonly occurs.

The student is usually given an active role in working up the patient and preparing him for surgery. The sense of concern and responsibility that the student develops for the patient in the first stage of surgical care must not be destroyed by a brusque

93

disregard of the student at operation. He should be given the respect that his commitment to the patient demands. There are several factors that must be considered to accomplish this. There is invariably competition between student and intern for proximity to the action. Unlike rounds in internal medicine, where many people learn from one case, only a limited number of people can see and participate in what happens in the operating room. Some time should be taken during the procedure to demonstrate pathology and technical points to both interns and medical students. A limited commentary by the surgeon as the case progresses lets the junior people know he is aware of them and concerned about teaching them. This critical exchange of education for physical labor maintains the bond between surgeon and junior assistants and cements the assistants' loyalty. When the surgeon goes home at night, he can sleep more soundly knowing that the intern on duty has been committed to the patient by participating and sharing in the operation. To address the problem of junior level competition, a fair distribution of appropriate tasks such as knot tying and order writing should be assured. The direct involvement of the surgeon with the welfare of every member of his team is an extension of the principle of paying attention to details.

The duties of the primary-level assistant are straightforward and often tedious. When retraction is required, the surgeon positions the instrument and adjusts the tension for the assistant to maintain. If possible, the assistant should see the exposure created by his effort and keep the field in view to ensure that he is not slipping from his original position. This is not always possible, and he may have to rely on instructions from the surgeon. When he is required to adjust without direct vision, the assistant must be especially aware of the delicacy of the tissue against which he is pulling. Sometimes the surgeon becomes too engrossed and forgets to offer periodic relief to assistants. It is entirely appropriate for the assistant to request a break and stretch cramped muscles at a noncritical moment.

The hypnotic effect of prolonged inactivity can sometimes lead to unconscious expressions of boredom like humming and squirming. These signs should alert the surgeon to allow a break in the mental and physical tension.

The junior assistant should not get the feeling that his surgeon would prefer him to be a mute robot with masochistic tendencies and physiologic adaptations for prolonged hardship.

Advanced Assisting

As training nears completion, the senior resident should approach the ideal of a surgical assitant described at the beginning of this chapter. The first principle for a good assistant is to respect the leadership and direction of the surgeon. Initiative and independent action are inappropriate liberties unless indicated by the surgeon. It is generally best to respond to the surgeon's actions with the proper follow-up move, letting him direct the action and set the pace. The ability to maintain this relationship becomes critical in an emergency situation. Rather than grab for a lacerated blood vessel, the good assistant remains calm while being alert to the surgeon's instructions.

The second key attribute of a good advanced assistant is the ability to see the pattern of the surgeon's approach to a problem and to anticipate his next move. When the surgeon isolates a vessel, the assistant automatically applies a clamp to one side; the surgeon follows by applying his clamp to the other; the scrub nurse has the knife ready to hand to the surgeon to cut; the assistant takes the tie held taut and ready by the scrub nurse and ties the ends; the surgeon controls the clamps; and finally the second assistant cuts the knot with the scissors he has been holding close to the operative site. It takes longer to write this sequence than it should take to do it if each move is anticipated.

A third important factor in the performance of the assistant is timing. Only one hand should be in motion in the field at any one time. When the surgeon picks up peritoneum with his forceps, the assistant is still. The surgeon than freezes while the assistant picks up peritoneum a few millimeters distant. The assistant holds his position as the surgeon readjusts his forceps to ensure that he is holding only the single layer of peritoneum (see Figs. 12.9 and 13.9). Finally both forceps are still as the surgeon's right hand moves to cut the peritoneum between the two sets of forceps. The feeling for when to execute the appropriate countermove produces a flowing continuity. A corollary of knowing when to move is knowing when not to move. In his eagerness to help the surgeon, the assistant must not abandon one task, e.g., providing exposure, in order to do another, such as tying a ligature.

The final skill that a good assistant practices is keeping out of the surgeon's way. If there is a choice between the surgeon or assistant seeing clearly, the assistant must keep his head out of the way and out of the light. The assistant also uses instruments in such way that his hands are as far out of the field as possible. In order to be effective, the assistant must be proficient in the manipulative skills described in the preceding chapters.

Assisting as an Instructor

There is no one set of rules that applies to this category; rather, there is a spectrum of approaches to be used. Helping and teaching a junior resident demands active direction and participation. Teaching a senior resident may require acting as an ideal advanced assistant and offering only subtle suggestions and reinforcement. The problems with this level of assisting are mainly psychological. During the course of training, there is a turning point for most residents that may be gradual or abrupt. Prior to this point they have not mastered all the necessary skills and require strong direction and reassurance in the operating room. After the transition there is a feeling that everything has jelled, and this feeling manifests itself in a sense of control in the operating room. At this point the budding surgical ego is very sensitive to any perceived interference with developing style and independence. It is important to recognize the onset of this stage and encourage the trend. At the same time the instructor must exercise enough subtle control to protect the patient from harm. It can be a nerve-wracking experience for the instructor.

As the resident `gains more confidence in his abilities and his ego becomes less fragile, it is easier and more pleasant to assist him. At times such a resident may choose a weaker attending surgeon as an assistant in order to experience maximal independence. This is not entirely bad in that it is a step toward finally being on his own. There are a few caveats, however. There is always more to learn, and the best teachers are the ones to seek out for assistance to this end. Independent privileges for a chief resident can be very beneficial as long as they do not result in teaching the junior residents to the exclusion of their contact with senior staff. In order for junior residents to learn the principles of surgery well, they must be taught by the best qualified people early in their training. If they learn to do things right the first time, they won't have bad habits to unlearn later.

If an attending surgeon feels there is an obvious mismatch between a difficult case and the competence of the resident assigned to it, the conflict should be resolved before the patient gets to the operating room. Conflict and strong emotion in the operating room are unprofessional and dangerous. It is the duty of the instructor-assistant to ensure that both teaching and good patient care can be accomplished with every case he scrubs on. The attending surgeon can assess the qualification of a resident he doesn't know well by discussing the case pre-op. The resident's depth of knowledge of his patient, the pathology, and the surgical approaches should be clearly defined. If problems arise during surgery that are beyond the ability of the resident, the instructor is obligated to take over for the sake of the patient and to worry about the resident's bruised ego later. The subordination of ego to the good of the patient is itself a part of good training.

Chapter 7

The Operating-Room Team

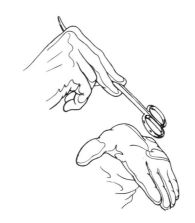

> *"But if another gives (the instruments), he must be ready a little beforehand, and do as you direct."*
> HIPPOCRATES (460–380 B.C.)

The surgeon is supported in the operating room by a group of people that functions as a team. The surgeon keeps open lines of communication with the components of the team and acts as the coordinator of the team's activity. The ultimate focus of all attention, including the surgeon's, is the patient. The team members carry out a sequence of coordinated steps. The circulating nurse organizes the preparation of the room while the anesthesiologist checks his equipment and medications. At the same time, the instrument nurse scrubs and organizes the instrument tables. When the anesthesiologist and circulator are ready, the patient is brought into the room and identification is confirmed. The chart is checked to make sure everything is in order. The circulator checks that the consent form is properly filled out and that the pre-op nursing checklist is completed. The anesthesiologist does a final check of laboratory reports and waits for the surgeon to make his presence known to the patient prior to the induction of anesthesia. The circulator and assistants oversee the transfer of the groggy premedicated patient from the stretcher to the table and secure the necessary restraints. If special positioning is required, it is usually done after the patient is anesthetized. The surgeon may help position the patient if the circulator is not familiar with exactly what is required. The surgeon and his assistants then scrub while the patient is being prepped. At the same time, the scrub nurse is completing instrument arrangement and preparing gloves, gowns, and drapes.

As the surgeon and assistants enter, the scrub nurse gowns and gloves them while the circulator observes for breaks in sterile technique. The scrub nurse hands the surgeon drapes, which the surgeon and his assistant place, again under the scrutiny of the circulator. Surgeon, assistants, and scrub nurse take their positions, and the cautery and suction are connected. Finally the surgeon checks with the anesthesiologist to make sure the patient is ready for the incision. Thus, the OR team consists of the surgeon and his assistants, the anesthesiologist, the circulating nurse and his assistants, and the scrub or instrument nurse. The function of the surgeon is addressed throughout the book, and the surgical assistant was covered in the preceding chapter. In the following sections the functions of the anesthesiologist, circulating nurse, and scrub nurse are briefly outlined.

The Anesthesiologist

The anesthesiologist (or nurse anesthetist) is a practicing pharmacologist. It is not possible to discuss the specialty of anesthesiology here, but it is important to understand the interaction that takes place between anesthesiologist and surgeon during a procedure. In addition to the practical aspects of giving his patient the best possible care und result, the surgeon is ultimately responsible for everything that happens to the patient in the operating room.

97

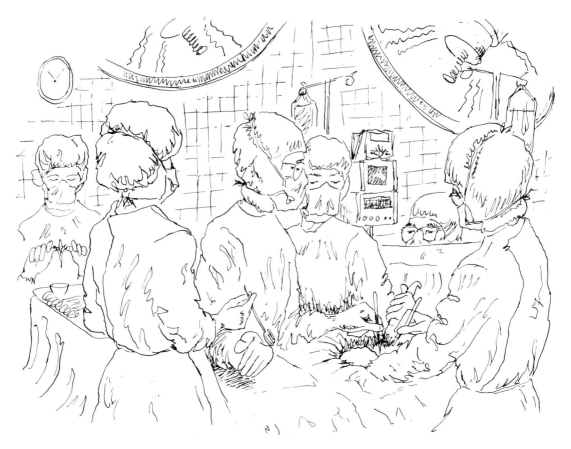

Fig. 7.1   The position of each team member determines the ease with which each can carry out his function. The table is at elbow height of the tallest person at the table. No one needs to stoop and develop back pain. For fine work the surgeon should wear magnifying loupes rather than bend closer. The second assistant (to the surgeon's left) is turned sideways to avoid crowding the surgeon. The first assistant stands across the table. The scrub nurse has clear access to pass instruments and see the operative field.

One light is directed over the surgeon's right shoulder and the other is overhead and cephalad in this case. If lighting is poor in a deep location such as the chest, the surgeon may opt to wear a fiberoptic headlight. The wide incision allows visibility and illumination and requires neither assistant to retract hard for exposure.

The attention of surgeon, assistants, and scrub nurse is on the operative field. The surgeon does not look up to receive an instrument. The instruments in use are long enough to keep hands out of the line of vision. The surgeon's right hand is the only one in motion. The second assistant has a clear view of what is happening and what he is retracting.

The anesthesiologist is keeping track of the progress of surgery, and the circulator replenishes supplies before they are missed.

Complete hair coverings are an aid to sterility.

In his pre-op evaluation of the patient, the anesthesiologist reviews the entire work-up. He is particularly concerned with factors related to anesthesia. Access to the upper airway may be affected by loose or absent teeth and the flexibility of the neck. The choice of anesthetic agent or method might be influenced by systemic factors such as cardiovascular disease or hypertension. Choice of agent could also be affected by drug allergy or inability to metabolize certain drugs because of liver disease or hereditary enzyme defect. Since he is responsible for maintaining blood volume during surgery, he confirms that an appropriate number of units have been typed and

cross-matched. He must also be aware of any fused bony structures in order to supervise positioning of the anesthetized patient.

During the course of the procedure, a mature, flexible relationship must exist between anesthesiologist and surgeon. Each communicates to the other the patient's status and the progress of the operation. The activity on each side of the anesthesia screen influences the other. Autonomic reflex caused by the surgeon's manipulation of the bowel may cause bradycardia. Lightening of anesthesia can cause spasmodic contraction of the diaphragm, which may disrupt a delicate part of the procedure. In certain extraordinary circumstances continual feedback and communication are essential – for example, the blood pressure monitoring and titration necessary during excision of a pheochromocytoma. Ego conflict that separates the domains above and below the anesthesia screen is inappropriate and dangerous.

Toward the conclusion of the procedure, anesthesiologist and surgeon work together to coordinate withdrawal of anesthesia so that the patient is not left with a large amount of muscle relaxant and anesthetic on board when it is time to wake up. The post-op respiratory care and the timing of extubation are the primary responsibility of the anesthesiologist but still must be done in close consultation with the surgeon.

The Circulator

Rarely during training are surgeons formally introduced to the responsibilities and concerns of the circulating nurse and scrub nurse. As a result the surgeon gleans only an incomplete picture of what to expect of the nurses and what they expect of him. The responsibilities are outlined in this and the next section.

After receiving and transferring the patient to the operating table, the circulator assists the anesthesiologist during induction. The circulator then sets up the lights and performs or supervises the patient prep. He oversees the gowning and draping and finally positions the instrument tables and connects cautery and suction. If he sees any breaks in sterile technique, he has the responsibility and authority to replace or resterilize the contaminated item. If there is the slightest cause, he is justified in ordering the patient reprepped and draped or the entire instrument table replaced. Because of the major delay incurred by such a change, it is wise for newcomers to the operating room to ask what is out of bounds and how they are expected to behave.

During surgery a good circulator remains in the room and available as much as possible. He keeps careful track of supplies and replenishes stocks before they run out. An important function of the circulator is to keep the surgeon and anesthesiologist informed of blood loss as measured by suction volume and sponge weight. He keeps a running count of sponges and needles with the scrub nurse. Labeling and dealing with specimens and cultures must be done accurately to avoid disastrous errors. While the circulator is doing all these tasks, he remains alert for threats to the sterility of the field, such as an observer leaning over the table or fluid soaking through drapes.

At the end of the procedure he runs sponge and needle counts. His report that the final count is correct is acknowledged by the surgeon. He assists with the dressing and coordinates movement of the patient off the table.

This brief description of the circulator's duties does not do justice to the complexity of his task. The reader is referred to the selected reading (Atkinson and Kohn, 1986) for an appreciation of the sophistication and technical demands of the operating-room nurse's job. There the reader will also find detailed descriptions of the sterile field, draping, and associated procedures.

The Scrub Nurse

The scrub nurse is the guardian of the sterile field as well as the provider of surgical tools. The hallmark of a good scrub nurse is his attention to the operative field. Rarely will his eyes deviate from the action in front of him. A second major attribute is the ability to anticipate what will be needed next. This quality improves with experience and familiarity with the individual surgeon's style. A new scrub nurse should be prepared by reviewing the technique before the operation. His instruments are organized in such a way that they are immediately accessible when requested. It is disruptive and exhausting for the surgeon to wait, ask for instruments one step ahead, or take his eyes from the field. A good surgeon may have a particular scrub nurse who always works with him. The attributes of a good scrub nurse are something like the attributes of a good surgeon, and the parallel is correct. The scrub nurse is a professional in a highly technical area.

There is some mystique surrounding the slapping of an instrument into the surgeon's palm. The placement is firm and definitive so that the surgeon knows the instrument is there, but it should not be forceful enough to bruise several metacarpals. The instruments are placed in a position from which they are easily shifted for use. The nurse positions himself so that he has a direct line of passage from himself to the surgeon's right palm (if the surgeon is right-handed). If instruments are passed around an assistant, the risk of contamination increases. The scrub nurse may position an instrument in a particular attitude according to the request of the surgeon (e.g., "points up" for a curved clamp). The scrub nurse should be able to match the length of the instruments to the depth of dissection. Instruments are often known by several names or eponyms that vary from place to place. A new team of scrub nurse and surgeon should coordinate vocabulary before the case starts.

As the case progresses, the scrub nurse cleans returned instruments and maintains the organization of the table. Particular care is given to handling and accounting for knife blades and needles to prevent injury and hepatitis.

The scrub nurse provides feedback to the surgeon by repeating the size of a suture when passing it and by stating the type of solution or medication pro-

vided. A running total of volume and concentration is provided when giving local anesthesia.

The sterility of the field remains the direct concern of the scrub nurse. Anything that falls below the table top or waist level must be discarded. Contaminated or wet drapes are covered.

Finally, the scrub nurse maintains a sterile instrument stand in case of emergency until the patient leaves the room.

Tension and excitement in the operating room are counterproductive. The instrument-throwing, tyrannical surgical "giants" are and should be a thing of the past. The interaction of a good OR team is calm and professional, and the operation flows smoothly as a result.

Chapter 8

Introduction to Staplers

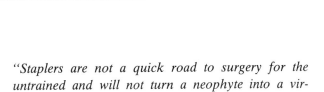

The evolution of surgical stapling devices occurred in parallel with the modern surgical era spanning the past 100 years. Now the training of a surgical resident would be incomplete if he or she did not become familiar with the advantages and pitfalls of using these instruments. While the importance of mastering basic principles of surgical technique is in no way diminished by the availability of these instruments, stapling is an important technical option. In experienced hands stapling results have proved equal or superior to hand-sewn suture lines in many applications, and there are unique benefits such as speed and access to remote anatomical sites.

This chapter is intended to provide the novice surgeon with an introduction to the development, structure, and function of modern surgical stapling devices. Facility in using these instruments can only be gained through hands-on practice, preferably, at first, in a formal stapler training course followed by supervised experience in the operating room.

Historical Development

During the last two decades of the 19th century, Halsted and other surgical pioneers developed the techniques that led to successful bowel suture and anastomosis. Almost simultaneously these same surgeons began experimenting with a variety of mechanical aids to improve the efficiency and results of their surgery. Halsted himself proposed an everting anastomosis effected by pressure necrosis between external cylinders apposed over an internal cylindrical stent. Many such devices were tried, and some established precedents for principles incorporated in modern stapling devices, particularly for the end-to-end instrument.

One of these early devices that gained widespread acceptance for clinical use and persisted into the 20th century was the Murphy button. This consisted of two mushroom-shaped halves. The stem of one half

101

fit snugly into the stem of the other with the aid of protruding spring ends and internal threads (Fig. 8.1). With the cap inside the bowel, the open bowel end was tied around the stem. The halves in the two bowel ends were pushed together, causing compression of the bowel between the cap rims. The central channel of the stems allowed immediate passage of gas and liquid stool. By the time pressure necrosis cut through the entrapped bowel after several days, the inverted serosal surfaces had suffi-

ciently bonded to maintain bowel integrity. The button then passed distally with the stool. An additional spring-loaded rim was used when anastomosing the thick-walled stomach. This anticipated the current principle of choosing the correct size instrument for the tissue thickness. The method of orienting the tissue for apposition is the same now used in the end-to-end stapler. Of course the tissue is no longer crushed but is left viable and held together by staples, and the diaphragm is removed by a circular knife.

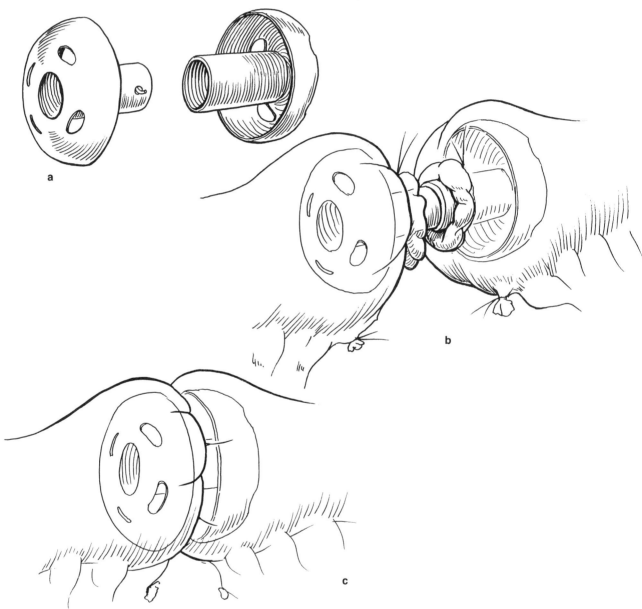

a

b

c

Fig. 8.1   The spring end protruding from the male stem of the Murphy button was pressed against the inside threads of the female stem to hold the halves together (a). The bowel ends were tied around the stems and the halves were mated (b). The apposed cap rims compressed the bowel walls, cutting out the enclosed tissue by pressure necrosis. By that time the serosal surfaces were sealed together (c).

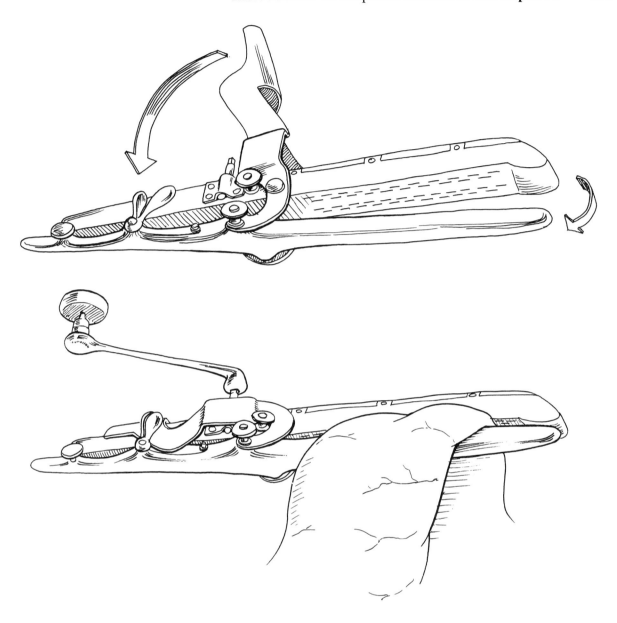

Fig. 8.2   Hültl's stapler drove individually loaded staples by a crank-and-pushrod mechanism.

The first true surgical stapler was developed by Professor Humer Hültl of Budapest in 1909 (Fig. 8.2). It delivered two double rows of fine steel wire staples, which were driven onto an opposing anvil to form a B-shaped closure. These same open-loop staples in modern instruments leave the microcirculation open to nourish the stapled tissue and allow normal healing, a fundamental surgical principle. Hültl's device, however, was complex, heavy, required hand-loading of the staples, and devitalized

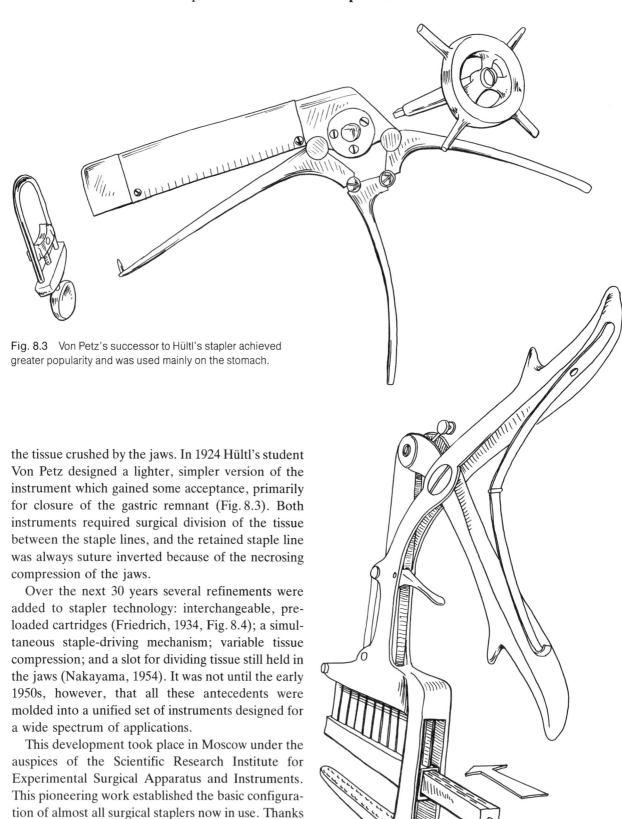

Fig. 8.3   Von Petz's successor to Hültl's stapler achieved greater popularity and was used mainly on the stomach.

the tissue crushed by the jaws. In 1924 Hültl's student Von Petz designed a lighter, simpler version of the instrument which gained some acceptance, primarily for closure of the gastric remnant (Fig. 8.3). Both instruments required surgical division of the tissue between the staple lines, and the retained staple line was always suture inverted because of the necrosing compression of the jaws.

Over the next 30 years several refinements were added to stapler technology: interchangeable, pre-loaded cartridges (Friedrich, 1934, Fig. 8.4); a simultaneous staple-driving mechanism; variable tissue compression; and a slot for dividing tissue still held in the jaws (Nakayama, 1954). It was not until the early 1950s, however, that all these antecedents were molded into a unified set of instruments designed for a wide spectrum of applications.

This development took place in Moscow under the auspices of the Scientific Research Institute for Experimental Surgical Apparatus and Instruments. This pioneering work established the basic configuration of almost all surgical staplers now in use. Thanks to the interest and experimentation with these Russian instruments by Dr. Mark Ravitch, an interest in stapling technology was generated in the United States, and further development was undertaken here beginning in the 1960s.

Fig. 8.4   Friedrich introduced the first stapler with an interchangeable cartridge.

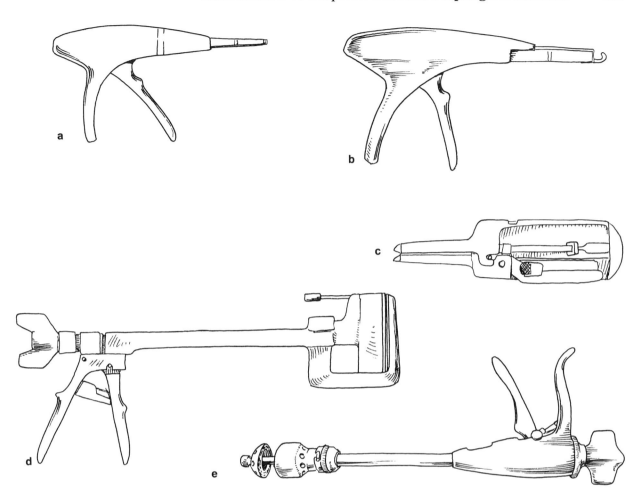

Fig. 8.5 Modern examples of the skin and fascia (a), ligating and dividing (b), gastrointestinal anastomosing (c), thoracoabdominal (d), and end-to-end (e) staplers.

Several goals were established to improve on deficiencies in the Russian prototypes. The American company that embarked on this endeavor, United States Surgical Corporation, set out to devise disposable, preloaded, presterilized cartridges to replace the hand-loaded Russian version, which required instrument disassembly for replacement. The new instruments were designed to be better balanced and lighter as well as simpler, with staple-driving fins and knife blades incorporated in the cartridge. A new category of instrument, the skin and fascia stapler, was added, and now disposable versions are becoming widely available from several manufacturers.

In the following descriptions of the various instruments, the illustrations depict the designs manufactured by United States Surgical because these are most widely distributed at this time and the operating principles and basic form are the same as for instruments more recently introduced by other companies.

Modern Stapling Instruments

There are five basic types of surgical stapling instruments (Fig. 8.5). The skin and fascia staplers insert successive individual staples to approximate incisions in those tissues. The ligating and dividing stapler places a pair of parallel hemostatic staples on an isolated band of tissue and divides between them. The thoracoabdominal group has the widest variety of uses, being applied to bowel, large vessels, and pulmonary structures (bronchi, lung parenchyma). These instruments produce a flat, everting closure. The gastrointestinal instrument is applied primarily to bowel for transection and anastomosis. The last type of stapler, the end-to-end anastomosing instrument, is especially beneficial when working in hard-to-reach locations such as the pelvis for a low anterior resection of the rectum.

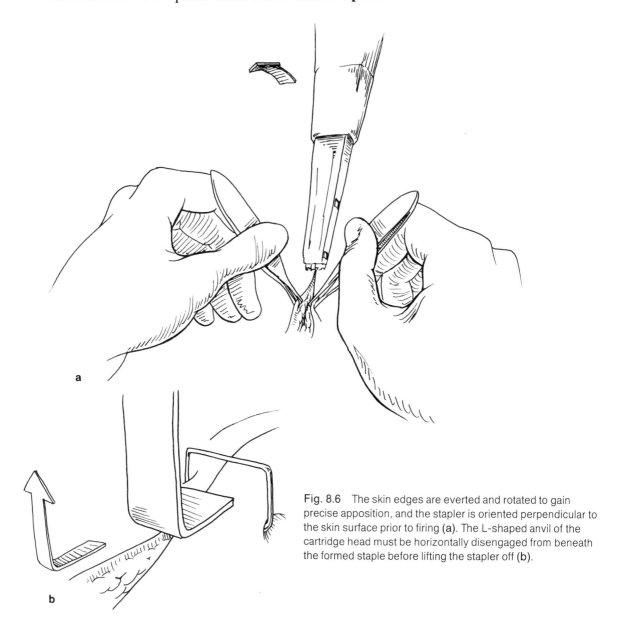

Fig. 8.6   The skin edges are everted and rotated to gain precise apposition, and the stapler is oriented perpendicular to the skin surface prior to firing (a). The L-shaped anvil of the cartridge head must be horizontally disengaged from beneath the formed staple before lifting the stapler off (b).

Skin and Fascia Staplers

These instruments are the most straightforward to use; the skin stapler has gained widespread acceptance because skin closure can be neatly accomplished in a fraction of the time required for hand suturing. The original reusable instrument took cartridges of 12, 25, or 35 staples, with a smaller staple for skin and a larger staple for fascia. The skin edges are apposed with slight eversion by the assistant while the operator centers and places the staple (Fig. 8.6). The rectangular shape of the closed skin staple maintains precise edge apposition. The fascial staples close to a flat "B" shape. The swivel head of the reusable instrument accommodates to the orientation of the incision. The disposable skin-stapling unit

(Fig. 8.7) has gained wide popularity, and a new gas-powered model has just been introduced. The skin staple configuration is designed to allow the transverse bar of the staple to "float" above the incision to avoid cross-hatching. Both staple placement and removal (Fig. 8.8) are relatively simple with a few minor fine points of technique: the reusable stapler should be precocked for steadier placement; the skin staplers should be withdrawn horizontally a short distance before lifting to avoid snagging the staple on the L-shaped anvil; there should be several millimeters of clearance between the surface being stapled and underlying bone or vessel; when removing staples, the crimping of the crossbar must be completed before lifting the staple out, to prevent patient discomfort.

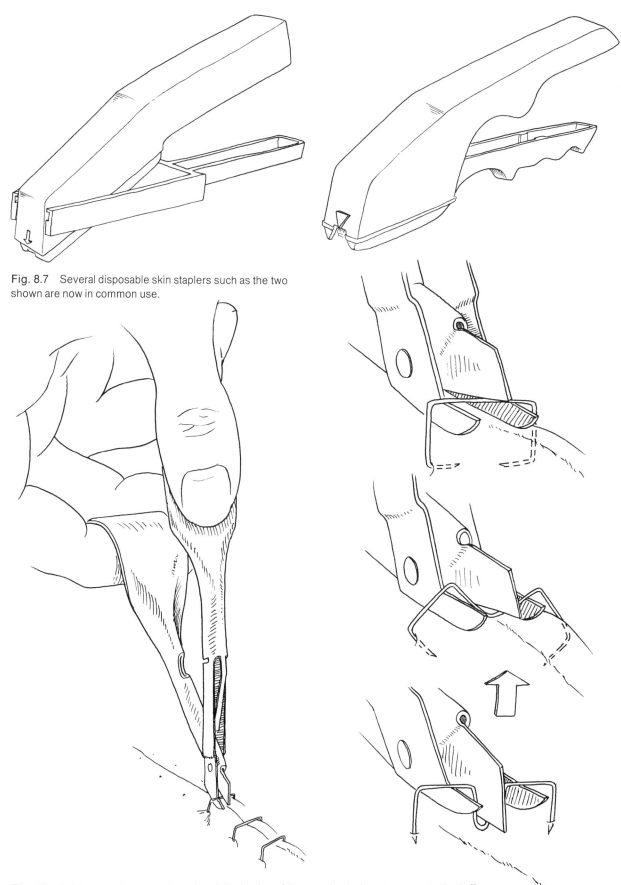

Fig. 8.7 Several disposable skin staplers such as the two shown are now in common use.

Fig. 8.8 Painless staple removal requires full crimping of the crossbar before the staple is lifted off.

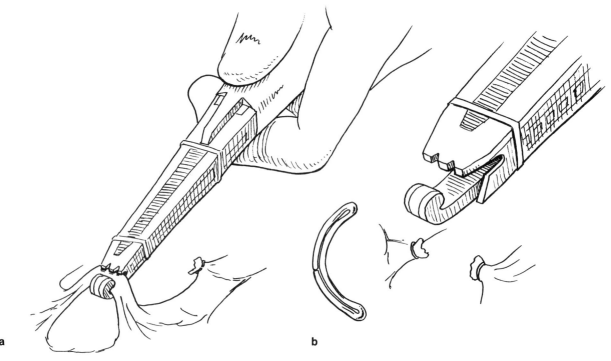

Fig. 8.9 The principle of avoiding mass ligature applies to the ligating and dividing stapler (a). The closed staples assume a crescent shape, and the tissue is divided between pairs of staples (b).

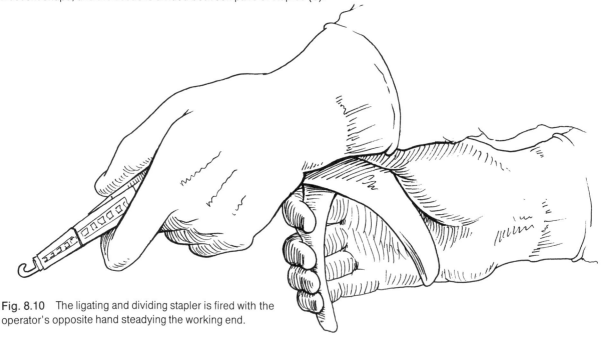

Fig. 8.10 The ligating and dividing stapler is fired with the operator's opposite hand steadying the working end.

Ligating and Dividing Stapler

The ligating and dividing stapler incorporates a hook-like jaw at the working end of the cartridge to hold the band of tissue to be divided (Fig. 8.9). The staples, which come in two sizes, are crimped around the isolated tissue in pairs. The closed staple takes the shape of a crescent. A central knife divides the clipped tissue at the end of the firing compression. When the last of the six or fifteen pairs of staples has

been fired, the mechanism locks to prevent division of unstapled tissue.

This instrument is especially useful and efficient for ligating a thin mesentery with multiple small vessels, such as the gastrosplenic omentum. It can also be used on other tubular structures such as the cystic duct, fallopian tubes, and vas deferens.

Because of the tendency to lever the instrument on compression, the operator must be careful to steady the instrument with his opposite hand (Fig. 8.10).

After firing, the instrument must be withdrawn downward to cleanly release the tissue from the mechanism. The most common problem with this device is the tendency for the operator to become impatient and include too much tissue in the jaws, exceeding the compressive capacity of the staples. The basic principle of avoiding mass ligature applies here. A drawback of staple ligature is that the staples are more easily dislodged than a hand-tied ligature. Rough manipulation or a carelessly withdrawn laparotomy pad can start significant bleeding. Major vessels such as the splenic artery should always be suture ligated for a safe closure.

Thoracoabdominal Staplers

These multipurpose instruments closely resemble Friedrich's stapler, which introduced the removable cartridge. An anvil compatible in size with the staple being used is placed on the terminal limb of the C-shaped outer jaw. The cartridge fits into the T-shaped inner jaw (Fig. 8.11). A pin is placed as illustrated to align cartridge and anvil and the wing nut brings the jaws together on the tissue. Vernier guide marks show the range of compression in which proper B-shaped staple formation will occur. Releasing the safety latch and compressing the handles drives all the staples simultaneously. If there is tissue to be excised beyond the staple line, such as a pulmonary bleb or Meckel's diverticulum, it is cut on the instrument while the tissue is still held firmly in the jaws (a reiteration of the basic principle that tissue must be fixed in position to be cut cleanly).

There are three sizes of thoracoabdominal instruments available, and they produce suture lines of 30, 55, and 90 mm in length. They each take a long-limbed (4.8 mm) and short-limbed (3.5 mm) staple; the use of each is determined by the thickness of the tissue. In addition, the 30-mm stapler takes vascular staples that are both smaller and finer.

The 30-mm instrument is primarily used for relatively small-caliber visceral structures such as small bowel and bronchus and for large vessels such as pulmonary arteries and veins. It is especially critical when stapling large vessels that the instrument be brought down to the tissue and steadied prior to firing so that no leverage or traction is applied that could avulse the structure. Such a vascular closure must be checked in case an additional fine suture is required.

The 55-mm stapler is used when a longer gastrointestinal closure is needed and for closure of larger

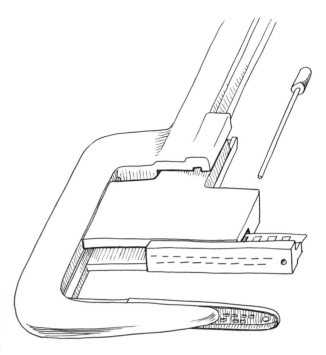

Fig. 8.11 The cartridge, anvil, and aligning pin are placed in the jaws of the thoracoabdominal instrument. The pin limits the lateral spread of the compressed tissue and keeps it within range of the staples. The staples take the shape of a "B."

pulmonary structures such as a main bronchus. The 90-mm instrument is most useful for resection of pulmonary parenchyma and for gastric work.

The disposable versions of these instruments now available incorporate design changes that may mean simpler and safer operation.

Some general precautions must be observed with all stapling devices. Cartridges and instruments must be checked for mechanical defects, usually resulting from improper maintenance. The more common cause of problems is improper use of the instruments. The stapled tissue must have an adequate blood supply, be free of disease, and be easily compressible within the defined range of the instrument and cartridge. Excessively thick or thin tissue should be hand sutured. All tissue to be stapled must be included within the jaws and unnecessary tissue must be excluded. All closures should be checked for significant bleeders that must be controlled. Because the staple lines of these instruments leave everted edges, such bleeders are easily seen.

There are numerous technical errors possible, and these are due to both forgetfulness and unfamiliarity with the instruments. Such problems as failing to lock the safety latch, using the wrong size anvil or none at all, failure to use the aligning pin, or forgetting to compress the handles can lead to unpleasant sur-

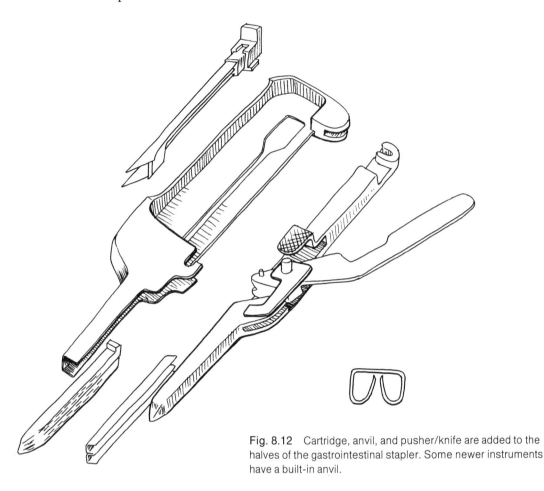

Fig. 8.12   Cartridge, anvil, and pusher/knife are added to the halves of the gastrointestinal stapler. Some newer instruments have a built-in anvil.

prises for the surgeon and morbidity for the patient. Meticulous attention to detail, another basic surgical principle, is the best defense against these problems.

Gastrointestinal Anastomosis Instrument

The gastrointestinal anastomosing stapler does what its name implies and also transsects bowel, leaving two closed ends. In addition, there is a cartridge without a knife blade for special purposes such as creating an ileal reservoir. In many applications this instrument is used in combination with the thoracoabdominal instrument, the latter closing the hole through which the former was introduced.

The instrument consists of locking halves that end in narrow beaks, one holding the cartridge, the other the anvil (Fig. 8.12). The two halves are partially assembled and then locked over the tissue to be stapled and divided. The activating mechanism consists of three long metal tines connected at one end by a plastic thumb tab. The center tine ends in a diagonal blade similar in shape to a No. 11 scalpel blade. The two outer tines successively drive the

staples in two staggered rows as the blade cuts between them. The staple-driving principle is the same one Hültl and Von Petz used in their instruments. The instrument is assembled as shown, with the three tines in their proper slots and the guide tabs on the pusher end seated in their own channel. After the pusher mechanism has been driven to its full depth, it is withdrawn and removed from the locked halves. The knurled release lever disengages the halves, which hinge open from the heel end and release the stapled and divided tissue.

This instrument, like the others, is subject to technical errors such as using the wrong size staples or an empty cartridge. Parts must be accurately assembled, and the tines and knife must be placed in the proper slots. If the instrument is difficult to close or fire, something is wrong. Uncontrolled wide separation of the halves while the jaws are still within adjacent lumina of anastomosed bowel segments can pull the anastomosis apart. Most surgeons using the instrument take the additional precaution of placing a suture at the distal end of this type of anastomosis where the staple lines end. The most significant

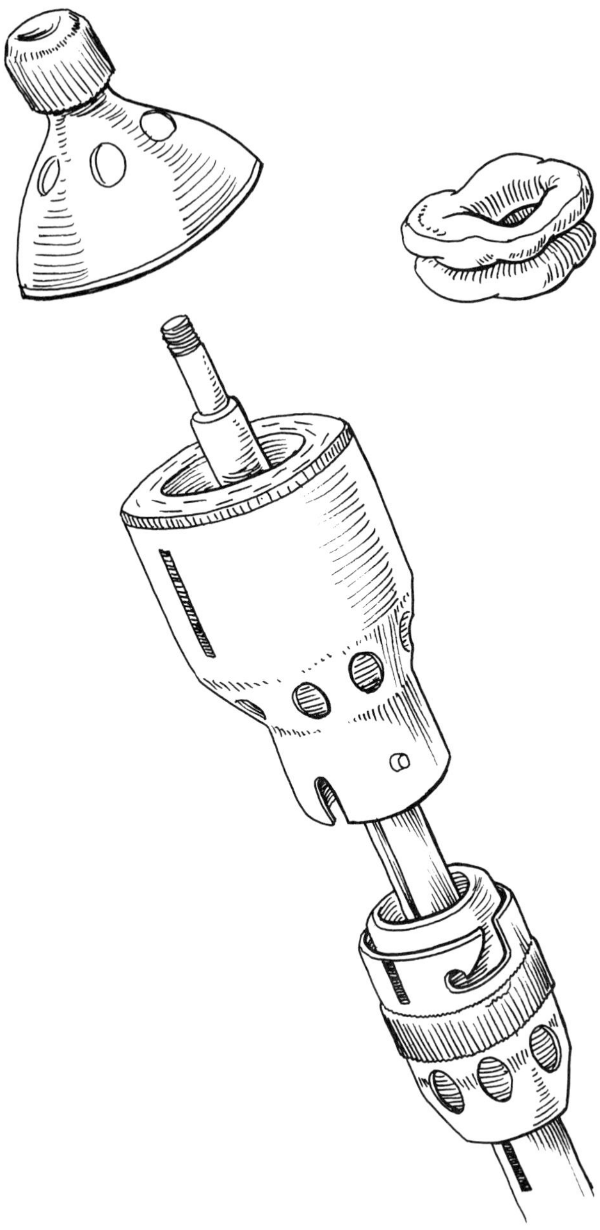

Fig. 8.13 The cartridge and anvil of the end-to-end stapler are placed on the shaft, aligned, and locked in position. Purse strings on the bowel ends are tied between the two, the safety catch is released, and the instrument is fired. After the instrument is removed and opened, the ring of excised bowel is inspected for completeness.

problem that can arise with this instrument occurs, ironically, as a result of its theoretical advantage: the ability to create an inverting anastomosis. Unlike the everted stapled edges created with the thoracoabdominal instruments, the internal anastomosed edges cannot be easily inspected for bleeding. Of course, when using the instrument for simply dividing bowel, this is not a problem.

End-to-End Anastomosing Instrument

This stapler is the most specialized and specific in its application (Fig. 8.13). It creates a circular, inverting anastomosis between two bowel ends. These ends are apposed by the same principle operative in the Murphy button and its successors. They are secured by purse-string sutures around the shaft between the nose cone and cylinder of the head. The purse strings can be placed easily and rapidly by using an ingenious purse-string clamp with a Keith needle (Fig. 8.14). After the wing nut approximates the head parts, the lever fires the staples and advances a circular knife. The cylindrical cartridge delivers two staggered rows of staples, and the knife cuts out the diaphragms created by the purse-stringed bowel ends. After opening the wing nut to separate the head components, one withdraws the bulbous head of the instrument with a gentle twisting motion. The instrument may be introduced through either a natural orifice such as the anus or through a lateral enterotomy, which subsequently must be closed. The end-to-end stapler is especially useful in the rectum when an anterior resection is low or the patient has a narrow pelvis. It is also useful for anastomosing esophagus and for connecting the stomach to an end lumen such as a roux-Y limb.

The usual technical pitfalls await the careless user, and there are special precautions that must be taken. The cartridge must be matched to the caliber of the bowel. Too large a cartridge can tear the bowel; too small a cartridge can leave a relatively stenotic anastomosis. The most serious problems arise when too much or too little tissue is included in the purse strings. In the former case the anastomosis may be distorted or damaged, and in the latter an incomplete anastomosis may result, leading to leakage and sepsis. The rings of tissue cut out by the knife must be inspected to make sure they are complete, indicating 360° of bowel end was between staple and anvil when the device was fired. The handles must be completely closed, as indicated by matching vernier lines, to ensure complete firing. The head components must

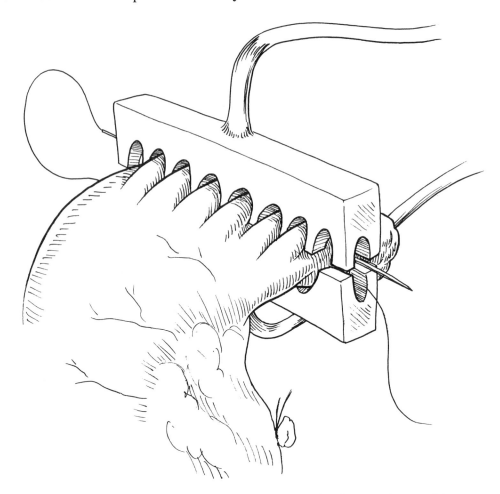

Fig. 8.14   Alternating ridges and grooves on the purse-string clamp create a complete purse string with two passes of a Keith needle.

then be opened by the wing nut to release the stapled tissue. Trying to withdraw the instrument prior to opening pulls the stapled anastomosis with it.

Summary

This discussion was meant to place the role of stapling devices in perspective in the context of modern surgical practice and to introduce some of their strengths and weaknesses. There are some situations in which the use of a stapler is unequivocally beneficial and other applications for which surgeons are divided in their preferences. The important point to remember is that these instruments are adjunctive tools, subject to all the rules that define the principles of good surgical technique.

Chapter 9

Microsurgery

David M. Lichtman

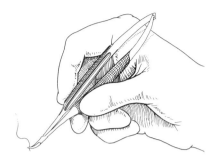

Historical Development

Two technical developments paved the way for the performance of successful microsurgery: the operating microscope and ultrafine suture material. The operating microscope was first introduced in 1921 when Nylen, an otolaryngologist, dissected the inner ear of a rabbit. Holmgren first used the microscope clinically in 1923 for the treatment of otosclerosis. Ophthalmologists initially utilized the microscope in 1946 for corneal wound closure and later for cataract surgery and the management of glaucoma. Kurze, a neurosurgeon, resected an acoustic neuroma in 1957, and in the 1960s urologists used the microscope for ureteral reconstruction. In 1960 Jacobsen coined the term "microsurgery" in describing the use of an operating microscope of up to 25 power to anastomose 1.4- to 3.2-mm animal vessels.

Dr. Harry Buncke began microvascular experiments in 1958 but had no success with vessels of 1 mm or less. Since the fineness of the suture material seemed to be the limiting factor, he had a 100-μ needle drilled and threaded with 15-μ suture. This resulted in too large a hole in the vessel wall. Next, in collaboration with Schulz at Stanford, he electroplated the ends of 7- to 15-μ suture strands to create a needle that was an integral part of the suture. Soon afterward, swaged microsutures became available from Germany, Australia, and Japan. This breakthrough opened the door for rapid development of microsurgical vascular and nerve repair as well as for musculocutaneous flap transfers. One of the most spectacular outgrowths of these advances has been the reimplantation of amputated parts.

Although modern techniques have yielded up to 95% success rates in some hands, anecdotal reports of successful reimplantation exist in the historical literature. The first recorded success is attributed to Fioravante who in 1570 retrieved the severed nose of a Spaniard, urinated on it to wash away the sand, and bound it back in place with balsam. Further success was recorded in 1625, when Molinetti, a surgeon, was credited with suturing a criminal's nose back in place after punitive amputation. In 1814 Balfour reported that an index finger that was replaced nonsurgically also survived. In 1962 Malt, at Massachusetts General Hospital, successfully reimplanted the right arm of a 12-year-old boy. This historic operation, although done without a microscope, focused the attention of the world on the tremendous potential of reimplantation surgery. There followed an explosive growth of microsurgery. Microsurgical technique has developed to the point where the totally amputated penis has been reimplanted; all functions have been documented in some cases.

Microsurgical Equipment

The tools of microsurgery include the magnifying apparatus, delicate instruments, and very fine suture materials. The environment in which these tools are used is critical to the success of the operation.

The environment should be quiet and relaxing. Sudden loud noises, active pagers, and noisy assistants detract from the quality of the work. The assistants must know the instruments and be able to pass them instantaneously upon request. This requires that the instrument table be properly set up and inventoried prior to surgery. The surgeon and assistant sit facing each other across a wide, hard board or a specially designed table with cutouts for their bodies (Fig. 9.1). The extended areas of the table on either side of the body support the elbows, forearms, and wrists, with the latter held in the pronated position.

Loupes and the operating microscope provide the necessary magnification and are available from several manufacturers. Loupes 3.2–5 power or more (Fig. 9.2) are used to prepare the tissue to be worked on. In the case of a reimplantation, the parts are inspected and debrided, and identifiable nerve and vascular structures are tagged.

Once the tissues are prepared, the operating microscope is brought into the field. The microscope may be ceiling mounted or on wheels, but the latter is less expensive and more versatile. The microscope should have a double binocular head with the ocular lenses 180° apart (Fig. 9.3). Fingertip focus and zoom controls are most convenient, but floor pedals are also satisfactory. The usual magnification range is between 6 and 40 power, and most work is done

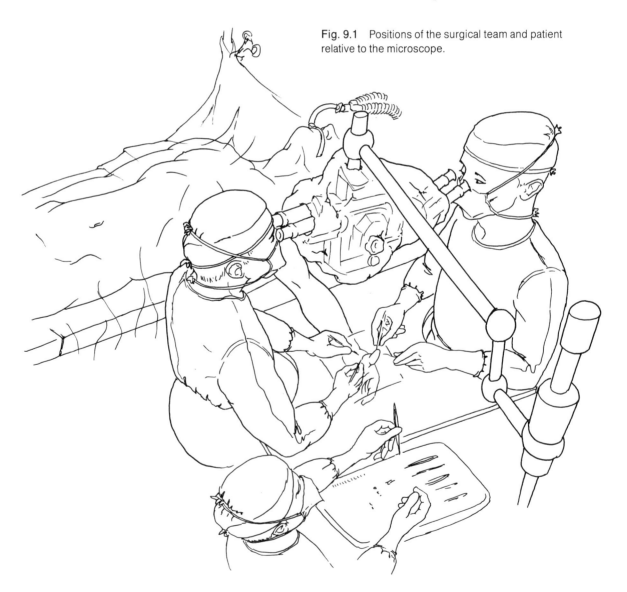

Fig. 9.1   Positions of the surgical team and patient relative to the microscope.

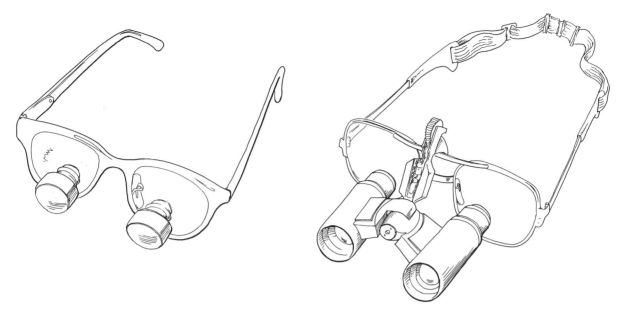

Fig. 9.2   Two examples of operating loupes.

using 10–24 power. Sutures are usually placed at about 16 power, but many surgeons lower the power to 10 while knot tying for the increased visual field. Higher powers (24–40) are used for close inspection (e.g., for intimal damage) and for checking suture placement. The microscope requires routine maintenance and careful inspection prior to each case. Extra bulbs should always be available. It is a good practice for the surgeon to sit down at the microscope with the assistant prior to scrubbing to focus the scope and adjust the eyepieces to suit their individual needs. A good supply of lens paper is also a necessity.

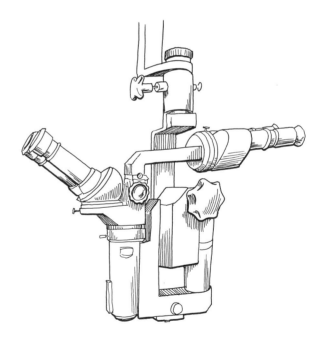

Fig. 9.3   Operating microscope with horizontally opposed double binocular head.

The choice of microsurgical instruments varies from surgeon to surgeon. The following is a representative selection comprising a basic instrument set:

1. A 13-cm round-handled, nonlocking needle-driver with straight (Fig. 9.4a) or curved (Fig. 9.4b) microtips.
2. A 13-cm round-handled, double-sharp microscissors with serrated edges and 9 × 2-mm straight blades (Fig. 9.4c), used for cutting vessels and microsutures.
3. A second pair of microscissors similar to the first but with curved tips, used for tissue dissection (Fig. 9.4d).
4. A 13-cm forceps with round handles and sharp tips, used for handling adventitia and tissue (Fig. 9.4e).
5. A second 13-cm round-handled forceps with curved, blunt tips and a tying platform (Fig. 9.4f), used for suture tying and vessel handling.
6. A third forceps similar to the second but with rat-tooth tips, used for handling more sturdy tissue (Fig. 9.4g).
7. A 30-gauge needle with the tip ground flat and turned to a 45° angle (Fig. 9.4h). This is attached to a 10-ml syringe with a Luer-Lok connector to produce a 500-μ stream of lactated Ringer's irrigating solution.

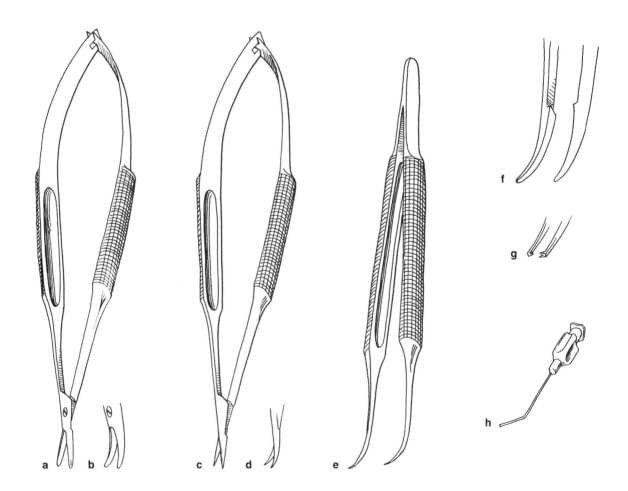

Fig. 9.4   a) A 13-cm nonlocking needle-driver with straight microtips. b) Curve-tipped needle-driver. c) Straight-tipped serrated microscissors. d) Curve-tipped scissors. e) Sharp-tipped forceps. f) Blunt-tipped forceps with tying platform. g) Toothed forceps for less delicate tissues. h) A 30-gauge, blunt-tipped, angled irrigating needle.

8. Microvascular clamps: We prefer double clamps mounted on a frame with a bar on which they can slide (Fig. 9.5). Suture-holding cleats are mounted on the frame. Two single Kleinert clamps are also required, with one having a 45° angle. An appropriate size clip applicator is used to manipulate the clamps.

The instruments are held in a three-point chuck pinch position with the handles resting on the index-thumb web space (Fig. 9.6a). The majority of microsurgical functions, including suturing and tying, are performed by slight pronation and supination movements of the fingers and forearm (Fig. 9.6b). Cutting is performed by a slight scissoring motion between the thumb and index finger (Fig. 9.7). When changing instruments it is best for the surgeon to continue looking through the microscope while the scrub nurse

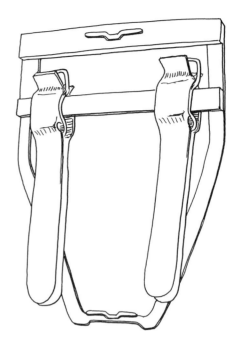

Fig. 9.5   Frame-mounted, sliding double clamps.

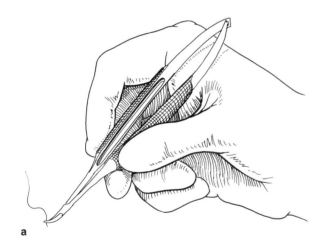

a

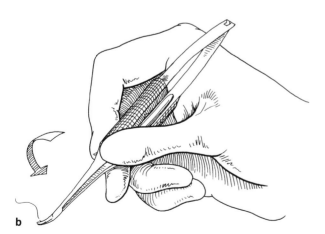

b

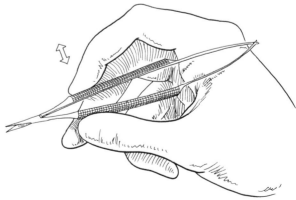

Fig. 9.6   Three-point chuck pinch position (a). Most microsurgical maneuvers involve slight pronation/supination movements of the fingers and forearm (b).

Fig. 9.7   Cutting involves a slight scissoring motion of thumb and index finger.

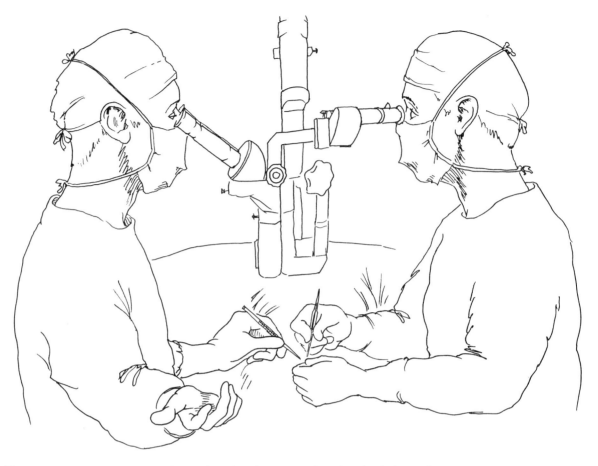

Fig. 9.8   The surgeon does not look away from the microscope when changing instruments.

removes and replaces the instrument in the surgeon's hand (Fig. 9.8).

There is a wide assortment of microsurgical needles and suture materials. The needles vary in both length and diameter. For general work one should keep on hand 8-0 and 9-0 nylon on 120-μ width needles and 10-0 and 11-0 nylon on 50- to 70-μ needles (Fig. 9.9). The latter will be useful for vessels under 1 mm, and the former will be used on 1- to 3-mm vessels and nerve fascicles. The needle curvature should be fairly shallow. There is sufficient latitude for individual preferences beyond these guidelines.

Finally there is a long list of relatively inexpensive but essential consumable or disposable drugs and equipment. Balloons of contrasting colors are useful for background material as is electrocardiograph paper, which provides a grid for measuring vessel diameter. Both, of course, must be sterilized. The two drugs commonly used are 1% lidocaine, for its vasodilating effect, and heparin solution, 1000 U/ml

of lactated Ringer's solution, to irrigate the ends of clamped vessels. An adequate supply of lactated Ringer's solution is needed to keep the operative field wet. A good supply of 2 × 2-inch gauze sponges and microtip sponge applicators are required to remove blood from the field.

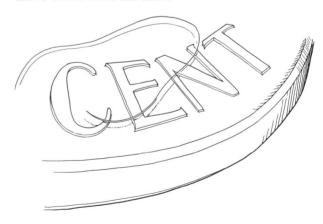

Fig. 9.9   The relative scale of a typical microsurgical suture.

Surgical Techniques

Basic Suture Handling

The three basic manipulations carried out on the microsuture are placing the suture, tying the knot, and cutting the strands. These are done using precise and controlled yet relaxed movements. Most microsurgery movements consist of barely perceptible (to the naked eye) pronation and supination of the hand-forearm unit and a rolling motion of the fingers. The best way to describe the movements involved in suture handling is by specific example. In the following paragraphs we use the placement of microvascular sutures for this purpose.

Under 10–16 power the lumen of the transected vessel end on the right side of the field is held open with the tips of the curved tying forceps, taking care not to damage the intima (Fig. 9.10). The needle is passed from outside to inside, perpendicular to the vessel wall supported by the forceps, and is passed through, following the curve of the needle with a supinating rotary motion. The point of penetration should be one or two needle-widths from the edge. The needle tip is passed into the opposite lumen under direct vision, taking extreme care not to catch either vessel wall. A gentle side-to-side motion of the needle will demonstrate if it is free of the vessel wall (Fig. 9.11).

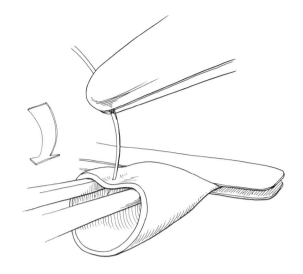

Fig. 9.10   The forceps supports the vessel wall while the needle is passed perpendicular to the surface.

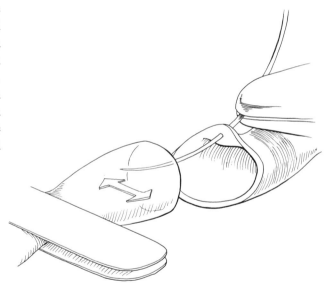

Fig. 9.11   Side-to-side motion of the needle tip demonstrates that it is free of the vessel wall.

It is best to advance the point slightly farther than required and then withdraw it to a point equal to the first puncture in its distance from the edge. With the tying forceps held open on the outside of the vessel to apply counterpressure, the needle is thrust upward following its curvature (Fig. 9.12). With the forceps still in place, the needle is pulled through from the outside using the needle-driver (Fig. 9.13). Without removing the forceps the suture is pulled through until only a short segment protrudes beyond the first puncture site. The long end of the suture attached to the needle is then curled like a "C," and the needle is placed on the colored background for easy retrieval after the knot is tied (Fig. 9.14).

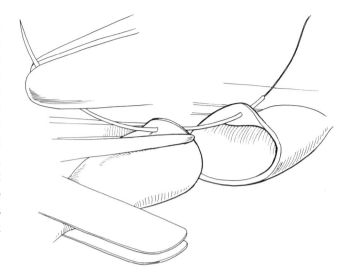

Fig. 9.13   With the forceps still in place, the needle is pulled through.

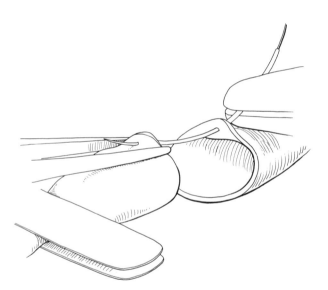

Fig. 9.12   The forceps provides counterpressure outside the opposite vessel end.

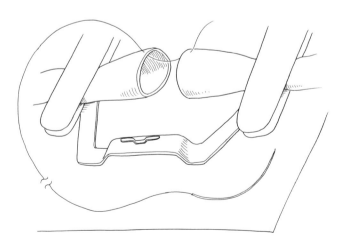

Fig. 9.14   The suture is curved into a "C" shape, and the needle is placed within easy reach on the colored background.

All knots must be square and tied with at least three flat throws. Ties in stay sutures should be started with a friction (surgeon's) knot and completed with three additional throws. The strands, of course, must be manipulated with instruments, and, with the modifications described below, the steps are similar to the instrument tie described in Chapter 3. Assuming the needle was passed from right to left by a right handed surgeon, the needle driver is in the right hand and the nonworking end attached to the needle is in the left. The tips of the forceps in the left hand are placed between the two strands from the far side of the vessel. This allows an easy forward movement to grasp the short working end, pushing farther into the loop so that it does not slip off the forceps. The loop over the forceps is formed by the needle driver crossing over to grasp the nonworking end on the left (Fig. 9.15). The throw is completed by drawing the instruments apart evenly, placing the strands opposite their starting positions (Fig. 9.16). The needle should not have been disturbed and should still be visible at the bottom of the field. The next throw is set up in the same manner, but now the needle driver is placed between the strands and the forceps crosses over to grasp the nonworking end (Fig. 9.17).

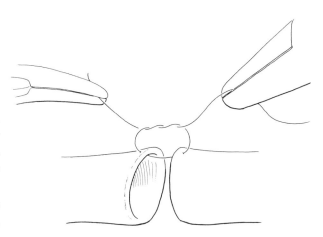

Fig. 9.16   The instruments are drawn apart to lay the throw flat.

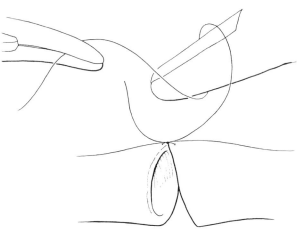

Fig. 9.17   The roles of the instruments are reversed for each subsequent throw.

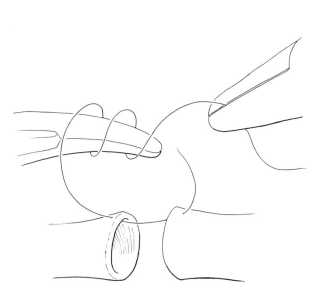

Fig. 9.15   The forceps is pointed toward the short working end and the needle driver crosses over to grasp and wrap the nonworking end.

The proper tension for the knots is sometimes difficult to judge with such delicate suture. In addition to one's "feel" or proprioceptive feedback, there is also a visual clue to the tension on the throw. When the light within the closing loop of the throw blinks out, the tension is sufficient and the knot will be secure (Fig. 9.18). Pulling beyond this point may break the fine suture.

The strands of the suture are cut individually, using the 13-cm microscissors with straight blades. The surgeon can cut them by placing the back of the scissors on the vessel next to the knot and slightly supinating the hand (Fig. 9.19a). This allows full visualization of the length of suture to be cut. The strand is then brought across the lower jaw of the scissors with the forceps (Fig. 9.19b) and the scissors are closed. The assistant may also cut the suture, using the same technique.

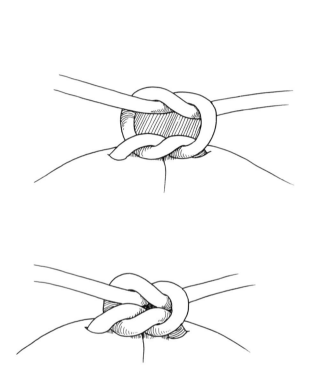

Fig. 9.18   The blinking out of the light within the knot is a good indication that proper tension has been achieved.

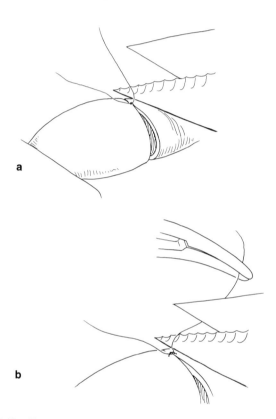

Fig. 9.19   The scissors are placed next to the strand to be cut and slightly supinated (a). The forceps bring the strand across the blade and the scissors are closed (b).

Preparation for End-to-End Arterial or Venous Anastomosis

After the cut ends are trimmed back to normal intima, a short cuff of adventitia is removed from each end to allow a clean suture line, minimize scarring and stricture, and relieve local vasospasm by sympathectomy. The adventitia is teased loose, pulled like a hood over the ends of the vessels, and cut flush with the vessel ends (Fig. 9.20). The remaining adventitia retracts back away from the vessel ends. This procedure is aptly referred to as a "circumcision

of the adventitia." If the vessel is in spasm at this point, the spasm can be relieved by bathing the vessel wall with 1% lidocaine.

Whenever possible a minimum of one artery and two veins should be indentified. If the intima at the cut ends of the vessels is not intact, the vessel must be debrided back to an intact area. Bone shortening or vein grafts can be used to make up for loss of vessel length. Vein grafts can be harvested from local tissue (e.g., the dorsum of the hand for finger amputation), but the surgeon must remember to suture the graft in the reverse direction to permit flow past any valves present in the graft.

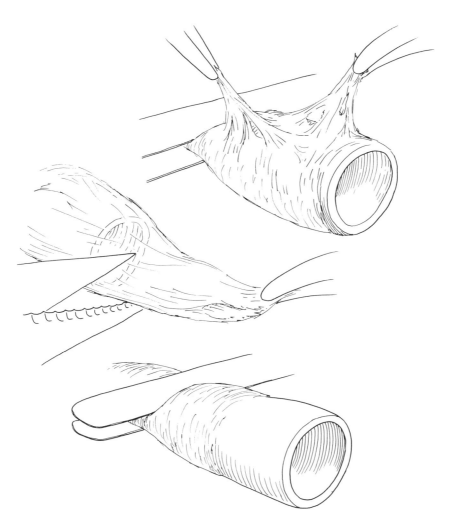

Fig. 9.20 The adventitia of the vessel end is teased loose, pulled over the end, and circumcised.

The vessel ends should be placed in the double clamps, using the clamp applicator to open the jaws and the blunt forceps to position the ends at the tips of the clamps (Fig. 9.21) to avoid torsion when the clamps are flipped 180° later in the procedure. The clamps now can be adjusted by sliding them together along the connecting bar to approximate the vessel ends without tension. The distance separating the vessel ends should be equal to the diameter of the vessel. If there is too much tension, feed additional vessel into the clamps one at a time. Persistent tension at this point must be corrected by vein grafting or bone shortening. After the tension has been adjusted, slide a square of rubber cut from a colored balloon beneath the clamp to provide a contrasting background. Light blue works well, but it is a matter of individual preference. Next, gently dilate the cut ends by spreading the forceps tips within the lumen. Holding the lumen open, carefully insert the tip of the 45° 30-gauge needle and irrigate out all clot from each end of the vessel using dilute heparin solution (Fig. 9.22). The vessel is now ready for anastomosis.

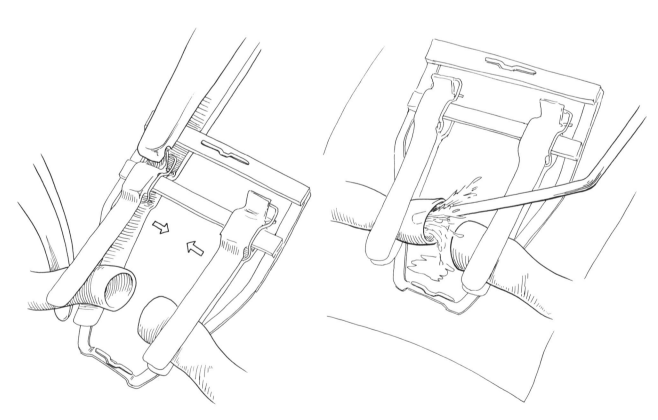

Fig. 9.21   The vessel ends are positioned in the double clamps.

Fig. 9.22   The vessel ends are irrigated with dilute heparin solution.

End-to-End Vessel Anastomosis

The method described here is one of several acceptable ways to reanastomose cut vessel ends and is preferred by many microsurgeons. This method involves triangulation of the vessel ends that are held within the aforementioned frame, which consists of two clamps on a sliding bar and a cleat attached to each end of the frame. For descriptive purposes we will consider the open end on one side in terms of a clock face, with the top of the circle closest to the surgeon being 12 o'clock. The first two sutures are placed at 10 o'clock and 2 o'clock and tied. One end of each is left long and wrapped around the far and near cleats, respectively, in an "S" shape (Fig. 9.23). If the cleat has been checked preoperatively and is clean, a gentle tug on the suture from the vessel side will demonstrate that it is securely held. These are stay sutures, and the tension on their ends will flatten the side of the vessel toward the surgeon and distort the clock positions, so those original positions must be kept in mind. After the ends are secured to the cleats, the first two sutures will now appear to be at the original 9 o'clock and 3 o'clock positions. The next suture is placed at 12 o'clock and tied (Fig. 9.24). If the vessel is under 1 mm, this completes the front wall suture line and both strands of the 12 o'clock suture are cut. For a larger vessel one end is left long to act as a stay while one additional suture is placed between 12 o'clock and each of the original stays (Fig. 9.25). The placement of these sutures is facilitated by the assistant gently pulling the 12 o'clock strand toward the opposite stay as each is passed. The central stay suture is then cut short and the front wall is complete.

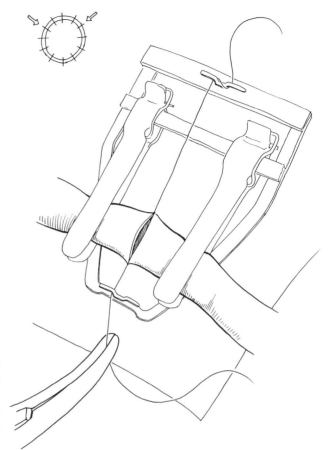

Fig. 9.23   The 10 o'clock and 2 o'clock sutures are placed, and a long end of each is secured to the respective cleats.

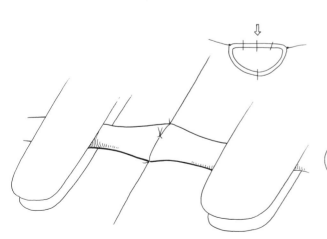

Fig. 9.24   The 12 o'clock suture is placed.

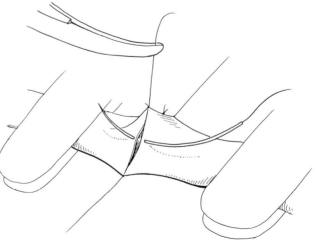

Fig. 9.25   For larger vessels, intermediate sutures are placed using the 12 o'clock suture to triangulate the vessel wall.

The frame is then flipped over by rotating the long side (relative to the vessel position) and stabilizing the short side to prevent kinking of the vessel (Fig. 9.26). Readjust the background material and recheck the focus at this time. The back two thirds of the vessel now faces the surgeon. Placing a central suture in the original 6 o'clock position triangulates the vessel by bisecting the facing two thirds. One end of this suture is again left long, and one or three sutures are placed between each set of stays, depend-

ing on the size of the vessel. If the vessel is over 1 mm and a total of twelve sutures is desired for the entire anastomosis, then stay sutures must be placed half-way between the primary stay sutures so that each segment can again be triangulated (Fig. 9.27). By this method a small vessel anastomosis will contain six sutures, and a larger vessel twelve. For intermediate vessels nine sutures can be placed in a similar fashion, by locating two equidistant sutures between each of the primary sutures at 10, 2, and 6 o'clock.

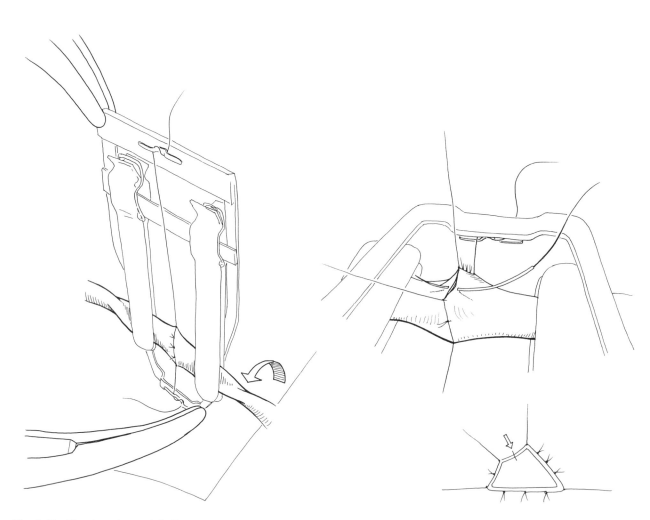

Fig. 9.26   The clamp is carefully flipped using the vessel as the axis of rotation.

Fig. 9.27   The back wall sutures are placed.

Completing the Anastomosis

After the last suture is placed, turn the clamp and vessel back to the starting position and release the clamp, which allows retrograde filling (distal for arterial and proximal for venous anastomosis) (Fig. 9.28). Unwind the stay sutures, but leave them long. After a few moments release the other clamp and cover the anastomotic site with some local fat (Fig. 9.29). Apply light pressure for a few minutes and then inspect the anastomosis. A small amount of bleeding is normal and will stop as the punctures seal with clot. If significant bleeding continues, carefully inspect the vessel to identify the site, reapply the clamps, and place an additional suture as necessary.

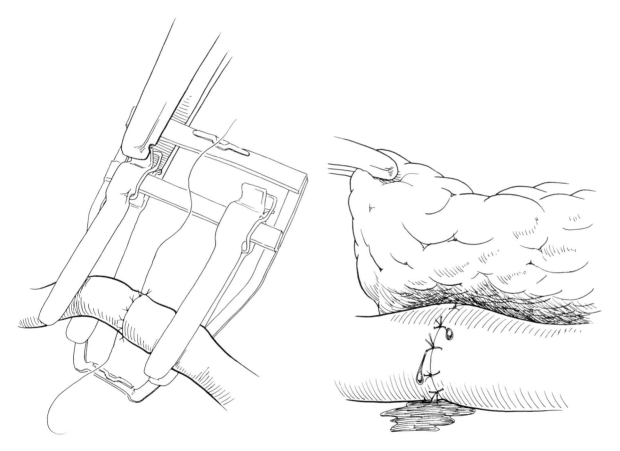

Fig. 9.28 The stay sutures are released, and the downstream clamp is opened first.

Fig. 9.29 Local fat is used to cover the anastomosis, and gentle pressure is applied until bleeding stops.

Although several patency tests have been described (downstream stripping [Fig. 9.30] and the flicker test [Fig. 9.31]), the true tests of vascular repair are capillary filling and venous outflow. These may be painfully slow to reappear because of vasospasm and must be awaited with patience and faith.

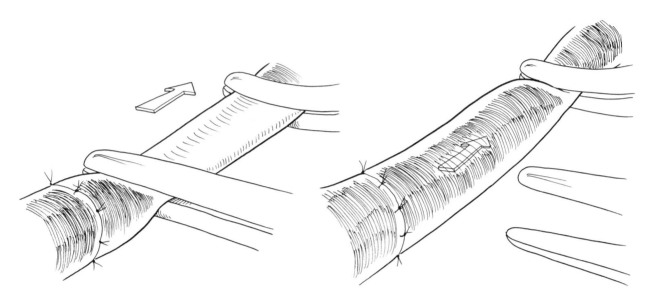

Fig. 9.30   The downstream stripping test demonstrates patency when the proximal clamp is released and the empty segment fills.

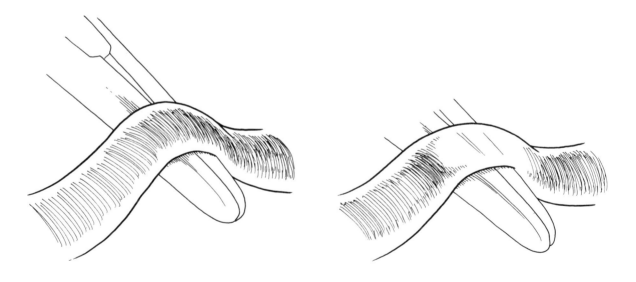

Fig. 9.31   In the ficker test, partial compression distal to the anastomosis results in systolic filling only and an alternating red and white flicker.

Summary

The discipline of microsurgery is an art as much as it is a science, and mastery requires diligent practice. The bare outline presented above is only an introduction. To gain functional microsurgical skills one must be immersed in an intensive lab-based training course (Fig. 9.32) and then put those skills to work on a regular basis. Patience and a steadied (vs. steady) hand are required, and self-control and self-assurance will come. Once mastered, the basic skills will persist, but periodic refresher training will hone those skills to an optimal level.

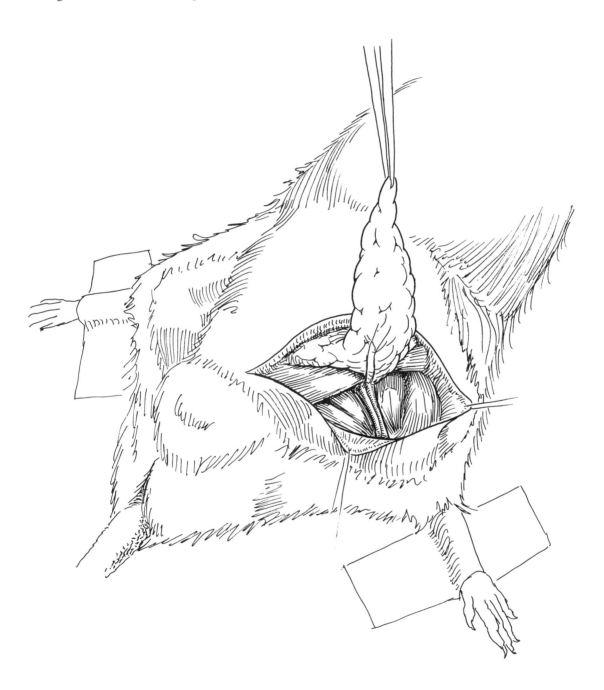

Fig. 9.32 The femoral vessels of the rat provide a good laboratory model for learning microsurgical technique.

Part II

Application of the Principles

"I believe that the tendency will always be in the direction of exercising greater care and refinement in operating, and that the surgeon will develop increasingly a respect for tissue, a sense which recoils from inflicting unnecessary insult to structures concerned in the process of repair."

W. S. HALSTED, 1913

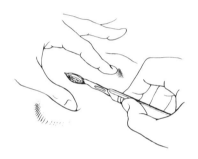

Part I analyzes the elements of surgery Halsted considered so important. The surgeon is the principal actor who synthesizes these elements to provide surgical care. The surgeon's knowledge of wound healing in particular must instill in him the "respect for tissues" that precludes "inflicting unnecessary insult." The personality traits we discussed promote calm and rational decisions and create a controlled environment in which the surgeon can exercise "care and refinement in operating."

The principles of asepsis, tissue handling, hemostasis, and exposure are the tools with which the surgeon achieves this goal. Manual skills such as knot tying and proper instrument usage can be developed with practice. Equally important for efficient surgery is the development of economical, purposeful movements – that is, the elimination of wasted movement.

The chapters in Part II are demonstrations of the principles in use. The surgical procedures are chosen to reflect the sequence of operations performed by the developing resident. In all examples but hernia repair, one method of performing each surgical procedure is selected. The chapter on surgical anatomy of the abdomen that precedes the abdominal operations shows certain clinically relevant relationships to stress the importance of anatomical knowledge. A fairly detailed anatomical discussion is included in the chapter on inguinal hernia because many find the surgery of this area confusing.

It is understood that the surgeon is thoroughly prepared for each of these procedures. Diagnostic workup and decision making, which are beyond the scope of this book, are the first steps. The surgeon must know the appropriate anatomy, pathophysiology, and alternative surgical procedures. The patient is fully informed and prepared psychologically and medically. Consultations are completed and technical arrangements for surgery are made.

We are now ready to operate!

131

Chapter 10

Minor Surgery

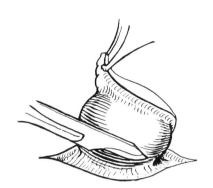

Minor surgery is predominantly concerned with dermal and subcutaneous pathology. The fact that a procedure is "minor" does not imply that it can be approached with any less respect than a "major" operation. The tendency to be less rigorous when doing a minor case often produces a bad result. If every procedure were done carefully with regard for principles and details of technique, fewer disfiguring scars would end up in the hands of the plastic surgeon.

All the principles of surgical technique apply to minor surgery. Careful tissue handling minimizes the dead tissue that is later replaced by scar. Inappropriately large or traumatic instruments kill large numbers of cells in proportion to the size of the incision. The skin hook gives excellent retraction with minimal tissue necrosis compared to an Adson forceps, for example. The presence of dead tissue, seroma, hematoma, and foreign material favor infection, which leads to more dead tissue and scar. The small scale demands precise hemostasis. Coagulating a vessel too close to the skin edge can cause a dermal burn.

Tissue response to surgical injury varies with age and body area. Scars in children tend to hypertrophy, and the fragile skin of an elderly patient may heal poorly. Scars subjected to movement during healing, such as those over joints, tend to spread. Certain areas, such as over the sternum, often produce hypertrophic scars. Careful technique and relief of tension help minimize the buildup of scar tissue.

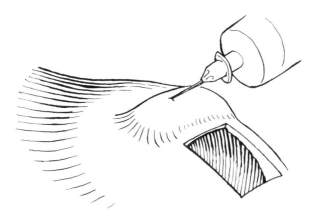

Fig. 10.1   The central area of the skin overlying most abscesses is thinned by pressure necrosis, giving the characteristic soft feel of fluctuance. The exceptions occur in the breast and buttock, where induration and tenderness may be the only signs of a deeper abscess. Probing with a needle helps localization in those cases. Injection of local anesthetic along the line of incision must be done very superficially with a fine (e.g., 25 gauge) needle. A minimal amount of local anesthetic should be injected to avoid adding pressure to the existing pain.

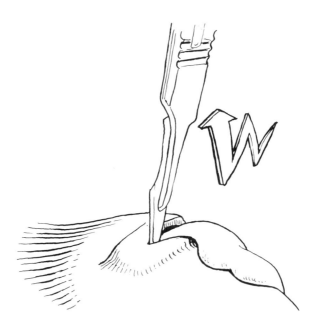

Fig. 10.2   Intradermal injection produces immediate anesthesia. A No. 11 blade is used with a sawing motion to make a wide opening.

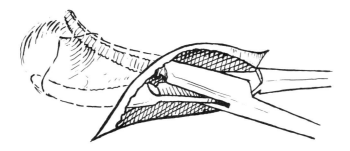

Fig. 10.3   The abscess cavity must be probed 360° around its circumference for loculations. This can be very painful in a large abscess. For breast and buttock, regional or general anesthestic in the OR is preferred to allow adequate exploration for loculations. Inadequately drained buttock abscesses are particularly prone to be complicated by spreading anaerobic cellulitis and necrotizing fascitis. Such abscesses should be treated under carefully controlled conditions, which only general anesthesia affords.

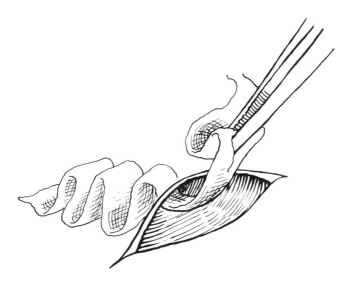

Fig. 10.4   The cavity is packed loosely from deep to superficial in accordion fashion for hemostasis in the first 24 hours. Thereafter, only enough packing is placed to allow drainage and to keep the incision open until healing closes the cavity from the bottom up. The packing may need soaking for easy removal on succeeding days. Less packing is put in as the cavity closes.

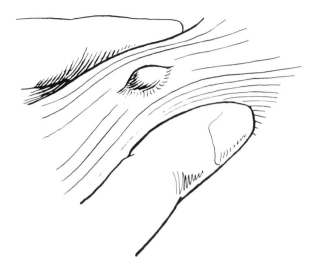

Fig. 10.5   If the skin is gently pinched in various directions, the stress lines will become evident. Incisions parallel with these lines heal with less scarring. These lines are generally perpendicular to the directions of muscle contraction.

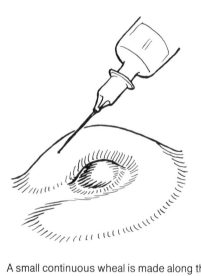

Fig. 10.6   A small continuous wheal is made along the proposed elliptical incision line. The needle is advanced to the hilt with each injection as the wheal is raised ahead of the tip, thus minimizing the number of sticks. Rapid stretching of skin causes pain; inject slowly.

Fig. 10.7 The incision is made with a No. 15 blade for fine control, and the heel of the hand is braced on adjacent skin. A No. 11 blade used with a stabbing motion produces even more precise corners. The ellipse should have a length-to-width ratio of greater than 4:1 to avoid dog ears at the corners. There are techniques for dealing with dog ears, but it is preferable to do it right the first time.

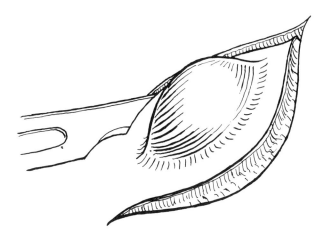

Fig. 10.8 The specimen is excised using diagonal cuts alternating from side to side. The depth of excision depends on the nature of the lesion.

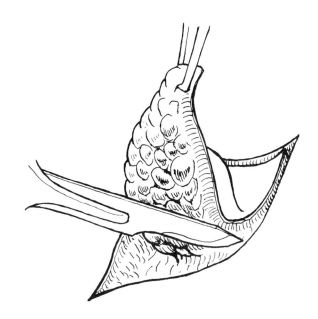

Fig. 10.9 The subcutaneous tissue is undermined, particularly at the corners, so that the edges can be approximated without tension.

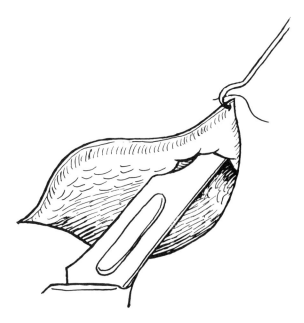

Excision of Sebaceous Cyst

Lymph Node Biopsy

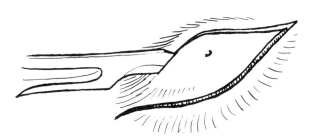

Fig. 10.10   The ellipse is placed around the punctum, which represents the gland from which the cyst originated.

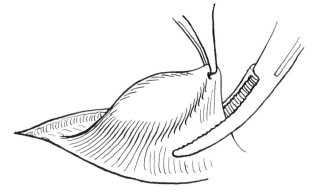

Fig. 10.12   The position of the lymph node is checked by repeated palpation as the dissection progresses. The areolar tissue at one end of the node is grasped for traction. Pressure on the delicate nodal tissue will cause it to fracture. The areolar attachments contain afferent and efferent lymphatics and are clamped or clipped to prevent a lymphocele.

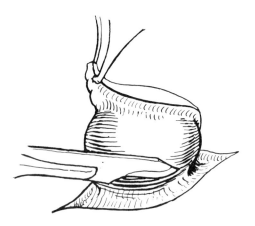

Fig. 10.11   The cyst is gently retracted and sharply excised. The entire capsule must be removed or the retained lining may cause recurrence. Cysts in dense skin such as the neck or back may need to be excised with a wider margin. The same is true of cysts that have had recurrent infection.

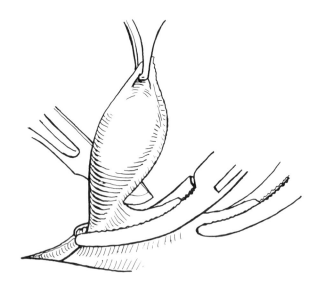

Fig. 10.13   The node is sharply excised and the lymphatics are secured.

Excision of Lipoma

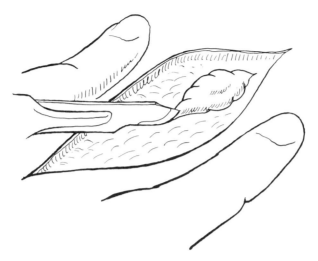

Fig. 10.14 Two fingers press on either side of the lipoma to localize and stabilize the lesion. The pressure also causes the lipoma to pout when the compressed pseudocapsule is incised. The lipoma is characteristically paler in color than normal fat.

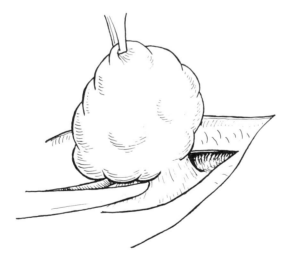

Fig. 10.15 If the proper plane is entered, the loose areolar attachments are easily divided, and the lipoma can be shelled out intact. Secure any significant feeding vessel.

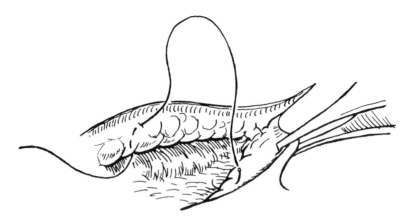

Fig. 10.16 Inverted sutures approximate the subcutaneous fascia to relieve tension on the skin suture line. The knots are "buried" away from the skin.

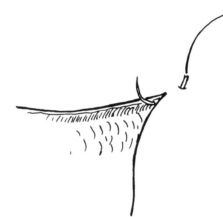

Fig. 10.17 Subcuticular sutures may be interrupted or continuous, absorbable or nonabsorbable. The first stitch of a continuous nonabsorbable subcuticular suture is passed into the corner of the incision just below the dermal-epidermal junction.

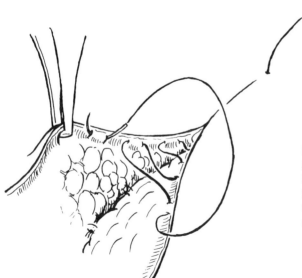

Fig. 10.18 Small horizontal bites of dermis are taken on alternating sides. The end is not tied, and the suture is left loose until the end of the run. The position of the next bite can be identified by pulling the suture across at right angles to the wound. The forceps gently holds skin immediately adjacent to each bite for control.

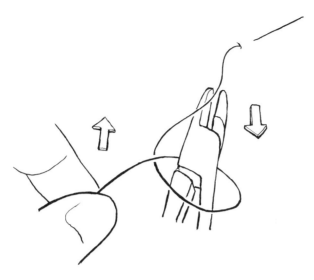

Fig. 10.19 When the suture line is completed, the suture is tightened by pulling the ends. An instrument tie is then done to knot each end at skin level. A loop is made around the needle-holder, and the suture is grasped about 1 cm from the skin.

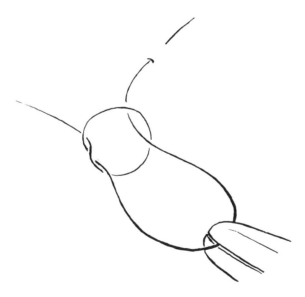

Fig. 10.20 The loose loop is then slid down to skin level and tightened. The process is repeated until the appropriate number of throws have been made. The wound may be covered with a plastic coating and/or paper wound-closure tape. The suture may be left in for a long period to prevent tension and spreading as the scar begins to heal.

If skin closure is done with penetrating methods, the sutures or clips should be replaced with adhesive strips by the third day to prevent cross-hatching.

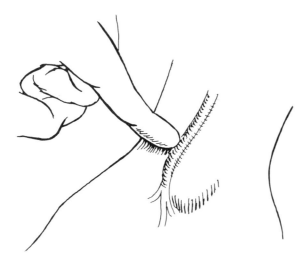

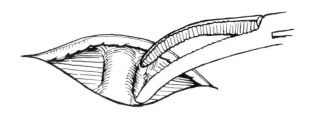

Fig. 10.23   The vein margin is defined on either side, and the clamp is insinuated between vein and bone.

Fig. 10.21   An emergency venous cutdown is most easily performed on the greater saphenous vein where it passes anterior to the medial malleolus at the ankle.

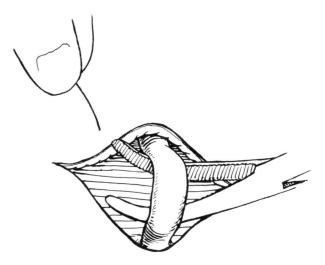

Fig. 10.24   The clamp is spread to obtain an adequate working length of vein. The small nerve that accompanies the vein should be left in situ when the vein is elevated. Proximal and distal ligatures are pased behind the vein.

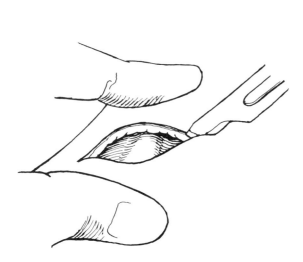

Fig. 10.22   Skin and fascia are incised to reveal the cordlike vein lying over the bone. The vein is invariably collapsed.

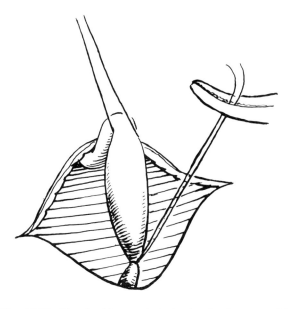

Fig. 10.25 The distal ligature is tied as far distally as possible, and the vein is elevated between ligatures.

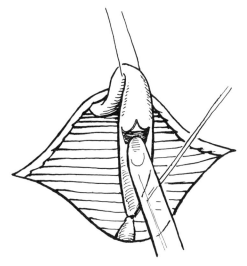

Fig. 10.27 A beveled, blunted catheter tip is placed in the opening with the bevel down. The catheter is gently inserted as tension on the proximal ligature is relaxed. Running some fluid through the line may help overcome spasm in the vein. A gentle twisting motion may also help thread the catheter.

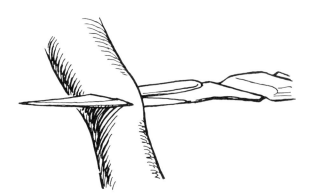

Fig. 10.26 At a point close to the distal tie, a No. 11 blade is stabbed through the center of the vein, with the blade beveled anteriorly and distally.

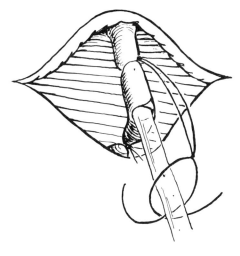

Fig. 10.28 The proximal ligature is tied snugly around the vein and catheter. A second knot is placed a short distance from the first, and the ligature is tied around the catheter itself. In elective circumstances the catheter can be brought out through a separate skin stab wound for sterility and ease of wound closure.

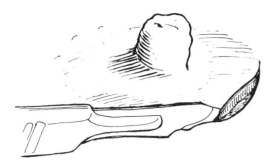

Fig. 10.29   If a benign breast lesion, such as fibroadenoma in a young woman, is within a short distance of the areola, a circumareolar incision provides good access and a cosmetic result. The skin is stretched to define clearly the areolar margin and allow a clean perpendicular incision.

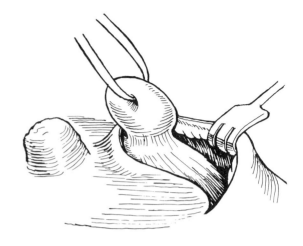

Fig. 10.32   When the lesion can be visualized, it is grasped. Fibroadenomas may fracture when grasped with a blunt instrument such as an Allis clamp. A traction suture or sharp breast (Adair) hook is more effective. The lesion can then be dissected from the breast tissue in which it is embedded.

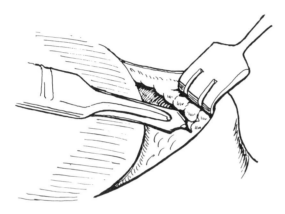

Fig. 10.30   The subcutaneous tissue is opened in a plane between fat and true breast tissue.

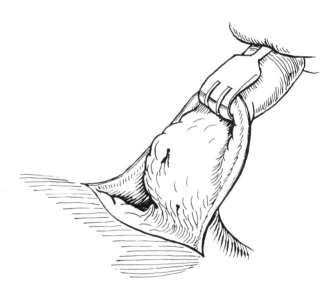

Fig. 10.33   The flap is inverted to achieve hemostasis. The depths of the wound are carefully examined as well. The cavity should be thoroughly irrigated. Breast tissue is extremely dense and must be approximated with a cutting needle and heavy (2–0 chromic) suture material. After the cavity is obliterated, the areola-skin margin can be reconstructed using a subcuticular stitch.

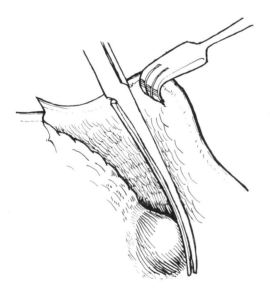

Fig. 10.31   The skin flap is elevated, and the lesion is palpated through each stage of dissection. Finger pressure from the skin side holds the lesion close to the incision.

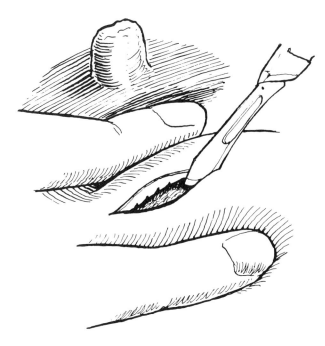

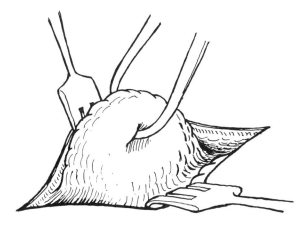

Fig. 10.36 The dome of the mass is grasped and elevated. Skin retractors are placed and finger pressure is released.

Fig. 10.34 The mass is localized between two fingers and held in place until it is directly transfixed with breast hooks. The incision is made in a manner that will not interfere with a subsequent mastectomy incision.

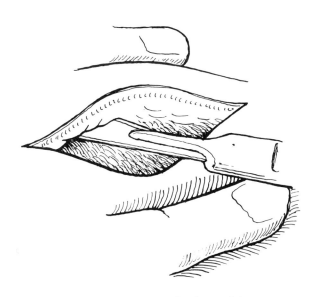

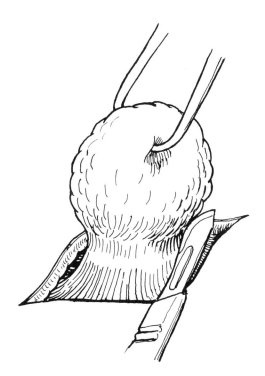

Fig. 10.35 Skin flaps are undermined around the circumference of the mass.

Fig. 10.37 The mass is sharply excised, with continued palpation to ensure an adequately deep margin. The margin depends on the purpose and philosophy of the surgeon. If minimal surgery followed by radiation is planned, a uniform, adequate margin is desirable. A wider margin can accomplish a virtual quadrantectomy, especially in a small breast. Even if the procedure is done strictly for biopsy purposes, an adequate margin ensures that the pathology will not be missed. The defect is packed with a sponge, and pressure is applied while the specimen is cut.

Chapter 11

Surgical Anatomy of the Abdomen

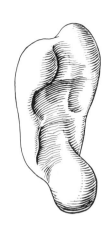

"Safety in surgery depends on knowledge of anatomy and technical skill."

S. HOPPENFELD, 1984

Abdominal Wall

The abdominal cavity is encased by a bony cap at its cephalad and caudad limits and is wrapped with a cylindrical girdle of muscle layers (Fig. 11.1). The lower rib cage, vertebral column, and pelvis protect much of the abdominal contents and serve as points of attachment for the encircling muscles. Posteriorly the vertebrae are supported by thick columns of the erector spinae muscles. The rest of the abdominal circumference is enclosed by the broad bands of the external oblique, internal oblique, and transversus muscles (Fig. 11.2). These muscles become aponeurotic anteriorly and form a sheath enclosing the long rectus abdominis muscles. The layers of the rectus sheath fuse in the dense midline linea alba. A layer of transversalis fascia lines the abdominal cavity and is separated from the enclosed parietal peritoneum by a layer of preperitoneal fat.

The cumulative power of the flat flank muscles is greater than that of the more noticeable rectus muscles, and may make transverse abdominal incisions less subject to distracting forces and dehiscence than longitudinal incisions. The alternating bias arrangement of these muscle fibers from layer to layer provides a secure, overlapping closure when the incision is made in the line of each layer's fibers. Retroperitoneal structures such as the kidneys and ure-

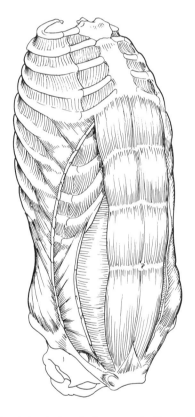

Fig. 11.1 The abdominal cavity is wrapped with a cylindrical girdle of muscle.

ters, great vessels, and sympathetic chains can be approached through the flank muscles without entering the peritoneal cavity. A short way below the umbilicus, the absence of aponeurotic fibers in the posterior rectus sheath makes the lower abdomen prone to incisional hernias.

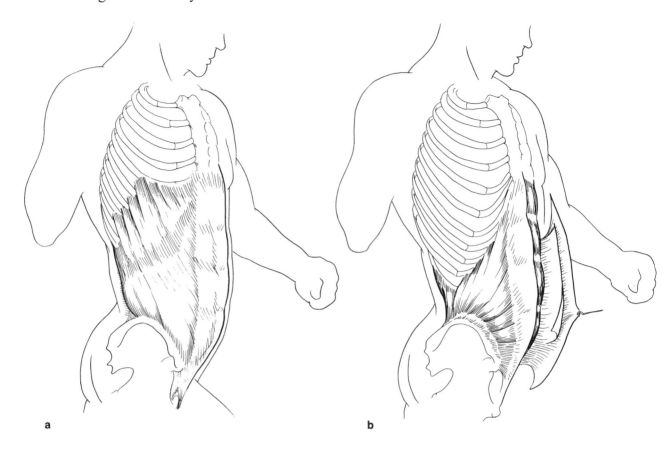

Fig. 11.2　a)　External oblique muscle. b)　Internal oblique muscle. c)　Transversus abdominis muscle.

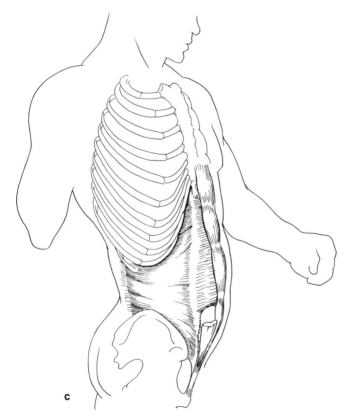

The vessels and nerves of the abdominal wall lie between the muscle layers; they supply the muscle and fascial layers and send branches that penetrate these layers to supply the overlying skin (Fig. 11.3). Familiarity with the segmental distribution of the lower thoracic nerves, which supply much of the abdominal skin, is important for neurological examination. Knowing that the tenth thoracic intercostal nerve terminates about the umbilicus, the anesthesiologist can assess the level of spinal anesthesia by testing for sharp sensation over the upper abdomen.

Within the rectus muscle the vascular ladder that unites the superior and inferior epigastric vessels has gained increasing clinical importance in recent years. It is now recognized that the majority of blood supplied to the skin comes from perforating vessels originating in the vasculature of the underlying muscles. By basing musculocutaneous flaps on one of the major muscular vessels, the surgeon can transfer large areas of viable tissue to distant defects.

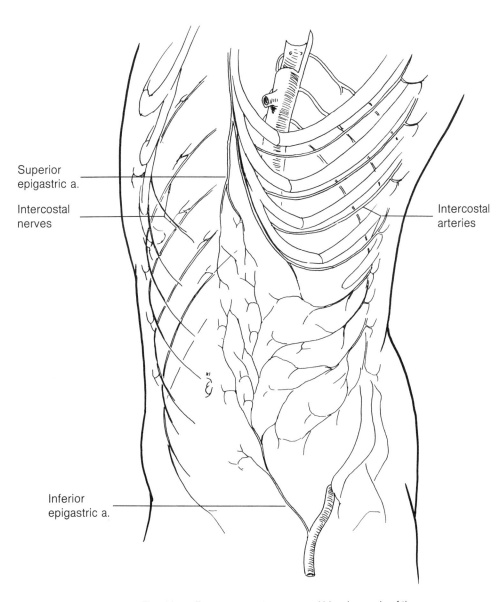

Fig. 11.3 The segmental nerves and blood vessels of the abdominal wall.

The posterior wall of the abdominal cavity consists of the vertebral column flanked by the psoas and quadratus lumborum muscles. The abdominal space is capped above and below by muscular diaphragms (Fig. 11.4). The diaphragm separating the abdominal from thoracic contents is perforated by three major structures: the esophagus, aorta, and inferior vena cava. The pelvic diaphragm has openings for the anus, urethra, and in the female, for the vagina.

The diaphragm provides the major power for quiet respiration and gently compresses the abdominal contents with each inspiration. Forced respiration calls into play the abdominal and chest wall muscles as well. The combination of forceful diaphragmatic and abdominal muscle contraction can dramatically increase intra-abdominal pressure. This is physiological in the case of defecation: the glottis closes and fixes the diaphragm in position while the abdominal muscles simultaneously contract. Such straining can also result from partial respiratory, gastrointestinal (left colon carcinoma), and genitourinary (prostatic enlargement) obstruction. Chronic increase in abdominal pressure puts stress on areas of potential weakness such as the esophageal hiatus and inguinal region and can initiate or aggravate hiatal and inguinal hernia. Obesity too can increase abdominal pressure, and all these factors must be considered prior to attempting the repair of a resultant hernia.

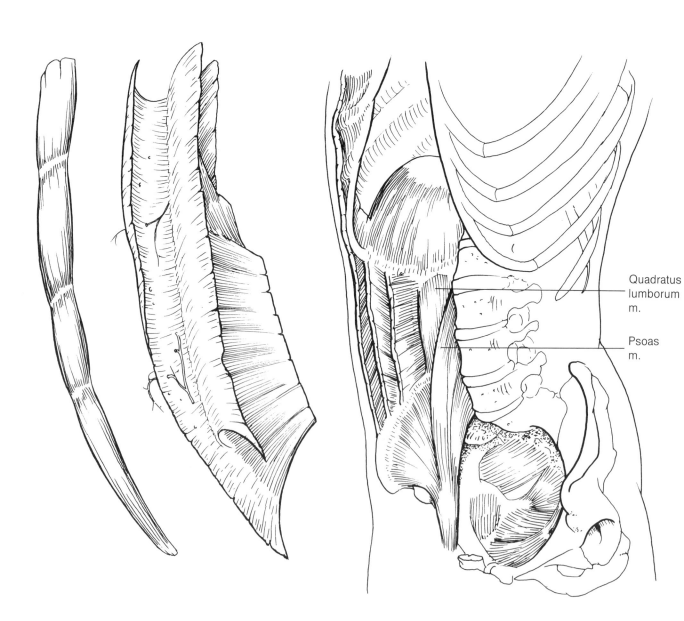

Quadratus lumborum m.

Psoas m.

Fig. 11.4   Posterior wall of the abdominal cavity.

Topographical Anatomy

The positions of the abdominal viscera relative to the body surface vary significantly from person to person and should not be rigidly linked in one's mind to bony or cutaneous landmarks. Within this range of variability, however, there are certain key relationships that should be noted because of their clinical importance.

If the skin were transparent on an anterior view of the torso, one would see a broad expanse of abdominal viscera extending from below the nipple line down into the pelvis (Fig. 11.5). The domes of the diaphragm may rise and fall a distance of two or three intercostal spaces, depending on the depth of respiration. Thus if a person were stabbed horizontally beneath the right nipple during expiration, the dome of the liver might easily be injured whereas during inspiration it might escape injury. The chest cavity overlaps the upper abdominal cavity almost down to the free edge of the costal cartilages. The lower limit of the pleura in the right costodiaphragmatic recess leaves only one or two interspaces through which to approach the liver for percutaneous biopsy or cholangiography without creating a pneumothorax.

Much of the upper abdominal contents, particularly the liver, spleen, and proximal stomach, are enclosed within the lower rib cage. In many instances this affords protection, but a blow forceful enough to break a rib can sometimes drive a jagged bone end into the highly vascular liver or spleen or at least rupture the capsule by the transmitted force.

The shape of the liver is variable, and the right lobe may extend well below the costal margin laterally. Palpation of the edge of the right lobe significantly below the midcostal margin usually indicates abnormal enlargement. Tenderness of the gallbladder when inspiration depresses it into contact with the examining fingers is sign of cholecystitis.

The angle formed by the costal margins at the xiphoid may be narrow or broad, depending on the build of the individual. A narrow angle may dictate that a vertical rather than a subcostal incision be used to approach the gallbladder. The popular subcostal incision offers good exposure, but it entails the division of two or three intercostal nerves, which causes numbness below the incision and partial denervation of the right rectus muscle. Unless an adequate rim of

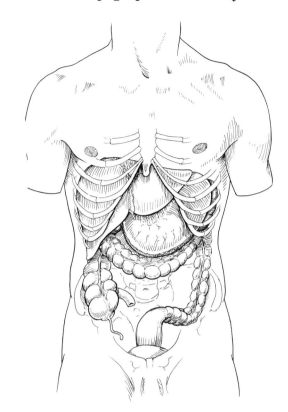

Fig. 11.5   Anterior surface relationships of the abdominal viscera.

flank muscles is left on the costal margin with this incision, a hernia may result that is very difficult to repair.

The mobile parts of the colon (transverse, sigmoid, and sometimes cecum) may be found in any part of the middle and lower abdomen. The vermiform appendix is particularly mobile, and inflammation of the appendix may irritate the rectal or bladder walls and result in diarrhea or dysuria.

The position of the bladder is relatively fixed behind the pubic symphysis, making it subject to injury from pelvic fracture. The dome of the bladder may easily extend to the umbilicus in obstructive uropathy. Such an enlarged bladder pushes bowel loops up ahead of it above the pubis, making suprapubic cystostomy by direct puncture safe to perform. Conversely, puncture for peritoneal lavage must always be preceded by bladder catheterization.

Small-bowel loops covered by omentum fill the remaining midportion of the abdomen, and their outline may become discernible through the skin if there is obstruction. The umbilicus corresponds to the level of the aortic bifurcation except in obese patients with pendulous abdominal walls. In thin individuals the distance between umbilicus and great vessels is remarkably small because of the vessels' position anterior to the prominent lumbar vertebrae.

The right lateral view of the abdomen (Fig. 11.6) shows the majority of the right lobe of the liver covered by the rib cage. The cecum is partially protected within the wing of the ileum. The upper pole of the kidney is normally found beneath the lower two ribs, but a ptotic kidney may descend all the way to the pelvic brim.

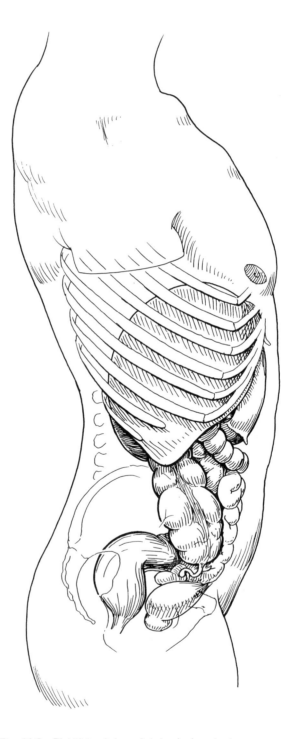

Fig. 11.6   Right lateral view of abdominal contents.

The left lateral view (Fig. 11.7) demonstrates the posterolateral position of a normal size spleen beneath the lower left ribs. When the patient is placed in the right lateral decubitus position, the tip of a slightly enlarged spleen may be palpated. The splenomegaly of myeloproliferative disease is easily palpated, and the spleen may occupy a large part of the upper abdomen. Note the flat profile of the lower abdominal contents, and correlate this with the cross-sectional anatomy that follows.

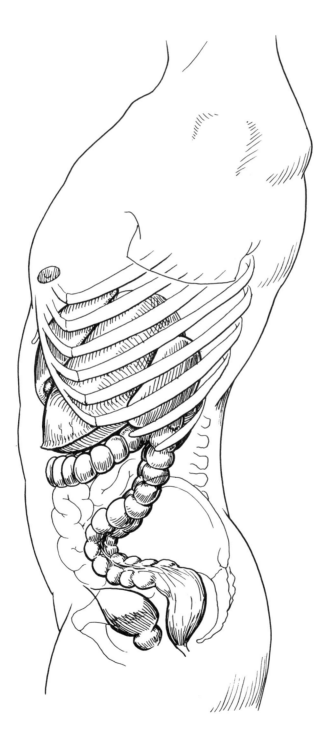

Fig. 11.7   Left lateral view of abdominal contents.

Cross-sectional Anatomy

The advent of computed tomography (CT) and magnetic resonance imaging (MRI) has made it more critical than ever for the surgeon to understand three-dimensional anatomical relationships. Although scan images can now be obtained in any plane and selected structures can be reconstructed by computer, a basic understanding of abdominal anatomy can be conveyed with a few cross-sectional planes. The level of the cuts is indicated on the key side views of the trunk. The sections are viewed from the caudad direction according to CT scan convention.

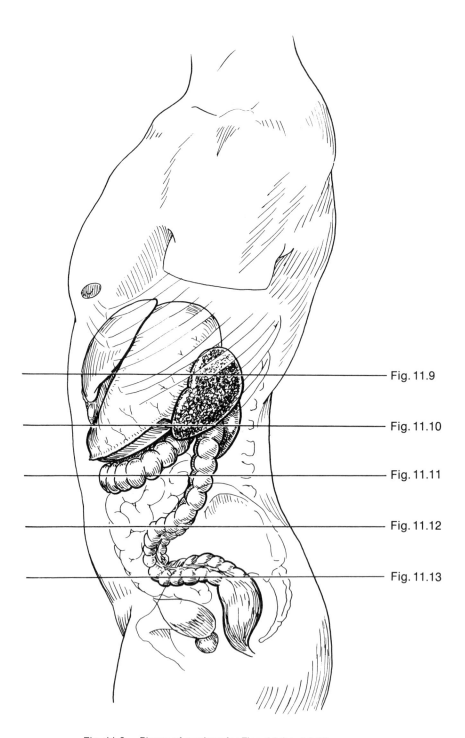

Fig. 11.9

Fig. 11.10

Fig. 11.11

Fig. 11.12

Fig. 11.13

Fig. 11.8.   Planes of sections for Figs. 11.9 to 11.13.

At the level of the xiphoid and the 12th thoracic vertebra (Fig. 11.9), the liver, spleen, and proximal stomach fill the domes of the diaphragm and are enclosed by the lower part of the rib cage (not shown). The hepatic veins drain into the inferior vena cava just cephalad of this section, and the adrenal glands are seen adjacent to the upper poles of the kidneys. The costophrenic sulcus is found external to the diaphragm along with a rim of the right lung. The esophagus has penetrated the diaphragm above and is opening into the stomach whereas the aorta is still posterior to the diaphragmatic crura. The tail of the pancreas is just caudal to this section.

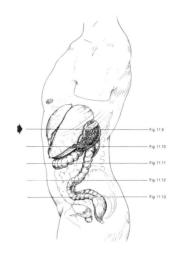

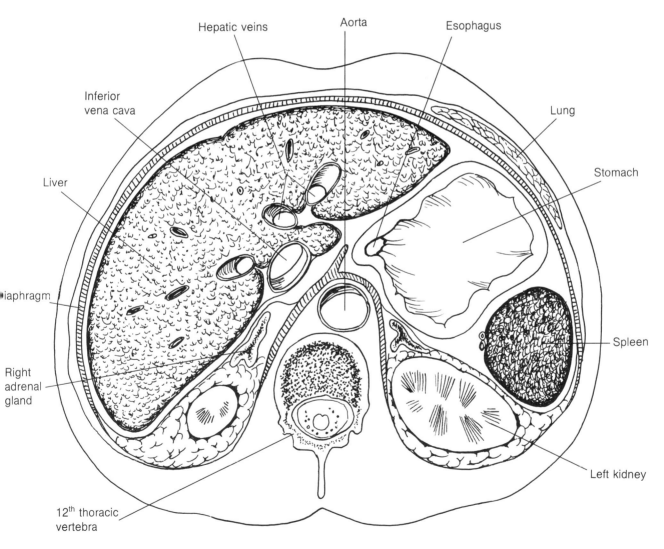

Fig. 11.9   Xiphoid level cross section.

The plane through the second lumbar vertebra (Fig. 11.10) bisects the right kidney and catches the lower pole of the left, as well as the lower pole of the spleen. The body of the pancreas, descending from the hilum of the spleen to the duodenum, is cut on the bias, as is the portal vein ascending toward the liver. Note that the pancreas is draped over the spinal column, bringing it close to the abdominal wall. In the short distance between the first two sections, the celiac trunk and superior mesenteric artery have already arisen from the aorta. The splenic flexure of the colon appears posteromedial to the lower pole of the spleen.

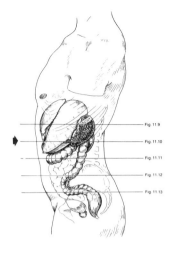

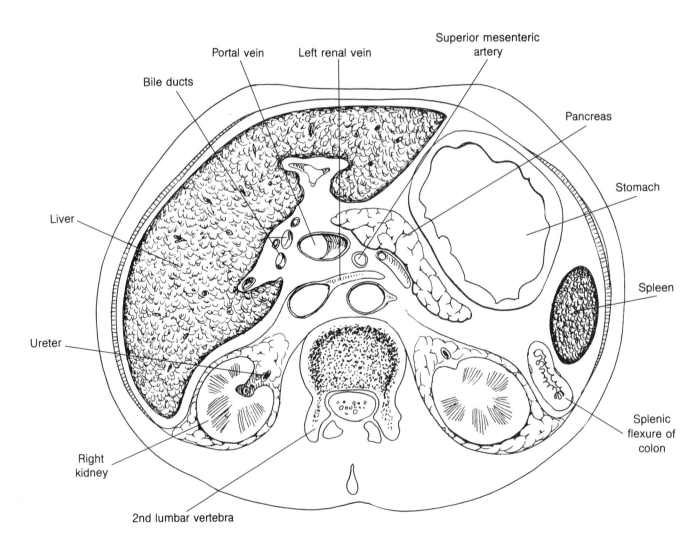

Fig. 11.10   L2 level cross section.

At the level of L4 (Fig. 11.11), the stomach in this patient has turned horizontally and disappeared from view while just the lower tip of the right lobe of the liver can be seen. Small bowel and omentum are omitted for the sake of clarity. We are just above the bifurcation of the great vessels, and the psoas muscles are becoming prominent on either side of the vertebral column. Note how low in the abdomen the third part of the duodenum is found and its intimate relationship with the aorta and vena cava.

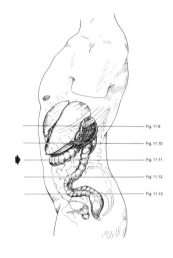

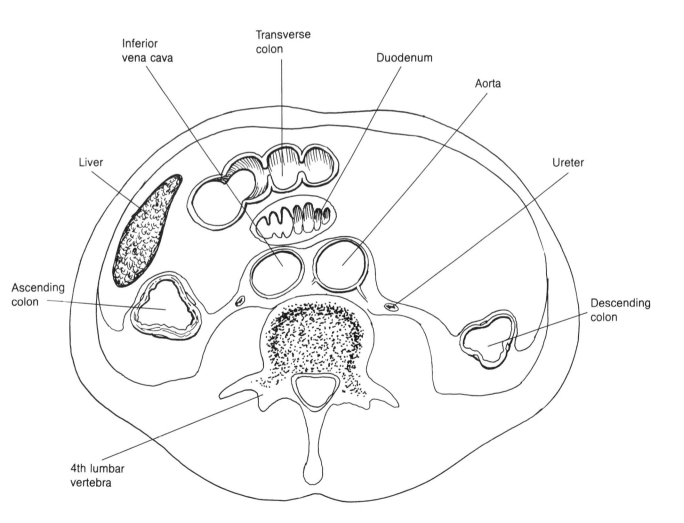

Fig. 11.11   L4 level cross section.

At the level of the upper sacrum (Fig. 11.12), the abdominal cavity has flattened out dramatically. The iliac vessels are diverging along with the psoas muscles on their way around the brim of the true pelvis to exit beneath the inguinal ligament. Note the contracted state of the small descending colon and the dilated ascending colon.

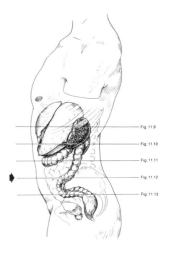

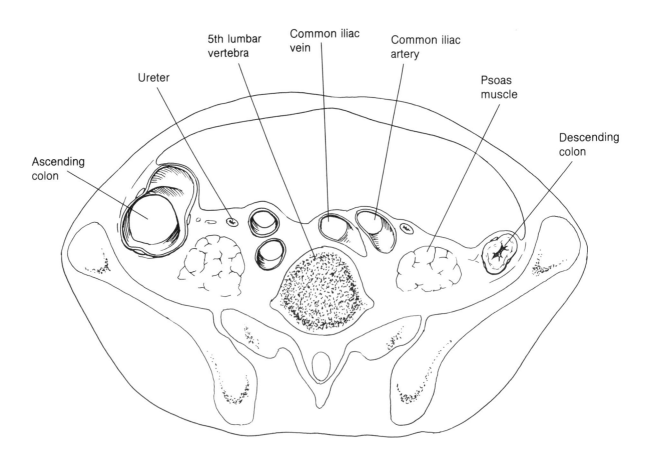

Fig. 11.12   Cross section at level of upper sacrum.

The final section (Fig. 11.13) traverses the true pelvis. The rectum has become retroperitoneal (approximately 4 cm of proximal rectum is surrounded by peritoneum). The ureters have crossed the iliac vessels and reached the lateral pelvic walls prior to turning anteromedially to reach the bladder. Caudal to this section the cul-de-sac between the rectum and the bladder/vagina marks the most dependent recess of the peritoneal cavity when the patient is in the upright position.

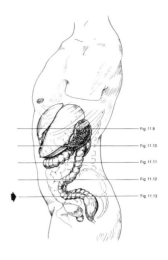

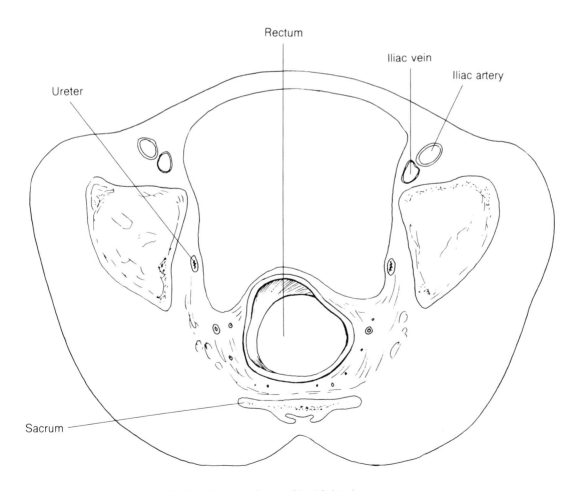

Fig. 11.13   Cross section at midpelvic level.

Peritoneal Cavity

The concept of the peritoneal cavity can be difficult to grasp. It is normally a potential space containing a small amount of serous fluid that lubricates the apposed parietal and visceral layers. It may expand with gas or fluid (blood, ascites, intestinal content) and become a true cavity under pathological conditions. The abdominal cavity contains both the peritoneal cavity and the extraperitoneal structures. If one focuses on the shape of the parietal peritoneum as the outer limits of the peritoneal space, interesting insights can be gained about the structures suspended within it.

The anterior view of the parietal peritoneum (Fig. 11.14) reveals the balloonlike cephalad expansions that fill the domes of the diaphragm. The lower abdominal portion is flat and broad whereas the pelvic extension balloons out posteriorly. There is one cephalad invagination around the ligamentum teres. In the lower abdomen there are vestiges of urachus and umbilical vessels along with grooves made by the inferior epigastric vessels (lateral umbilical folds). The anterior pelvic contour is indented in proportion to the distension of the bladder.

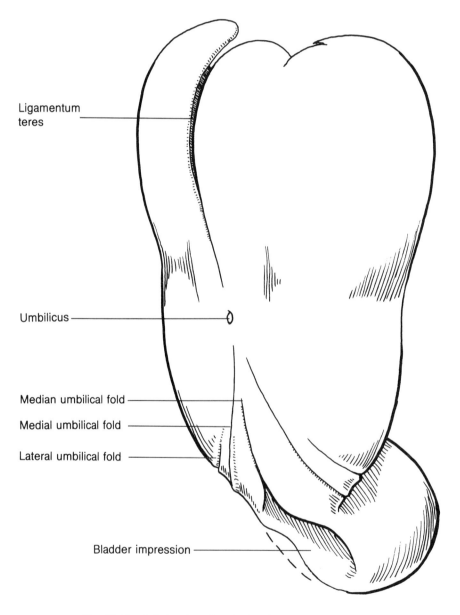

Ligamentum teres

Umbilicus

Median umbilical fold

Medial umbilical fold

Lateral umbilical fold

Bladder impression

Fig. 11.14   Anterior view of parietal peritoneum.

When viewed posteriorly the shape of the parietal peritoneum is much more complex (Fig. 11.15). There are numerous reflections, some of them named (e.g., the triangular ligaments of the liver). The broad attached areas of the right and left colon and rectum contrast with the narrow roots of the transverse mesocolon and small-bowel mesentery. Impressions made by the great vessels, pancreas, and kidneys shape the remaining surface. The constriction at the neck of the pelvic portion is accentuated by the yoke of the psoas muscles.

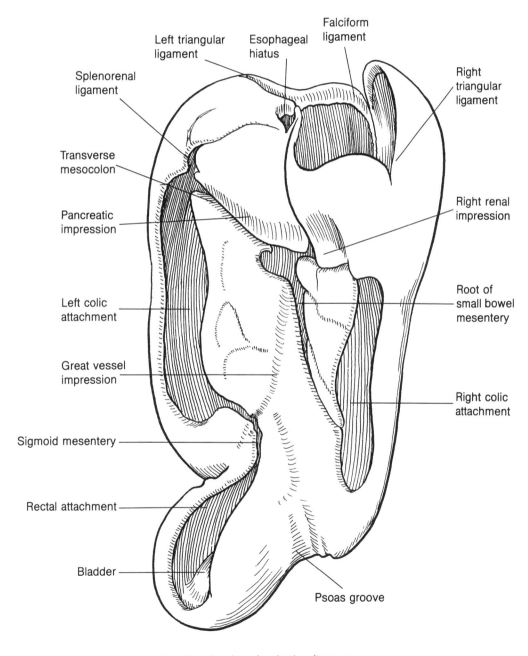

Fig. 11.15   Posterior view of parietal peritoneum.

Upper Abdominal Organs

Scanning technology has given us a fresh perspective on regional anatomy in contrast to conventional anatomical views. When the upper abdominal organs are viewed from a caudal direction, the first thing that strikes the observer is the dramatic crescent shape of the viscera draped over the spinal column (Fig. 11.16). The organs nest together compactly within the shell of the lower rib cage. In this view one can clearly see that the recess between the right kidney and liver is the most dependent point in the upper abdomen when the patient is supine; it is thus a likely site for subphrenic abscess. The proximal portion of the stomach lies in a more dorsal plane than the antrum, which is displaced anteriorly by the vertebral column. As a result, contrast material pools in the proximal stomach when the patient is supine and in the distal stomach when the patient is prone and upright during an upper gastrointestinal series. One sees the far posterolateral position of the spleen, which can make access tricky. The pancreas is draped over the vertebral column and is separated by only a short distance from the anterior abdominal wall, making it vulnerable to crush injury from an anterior blow.

Fig. 11.16   Exploded view of upper abdominal organs seen from a caudal perspective.

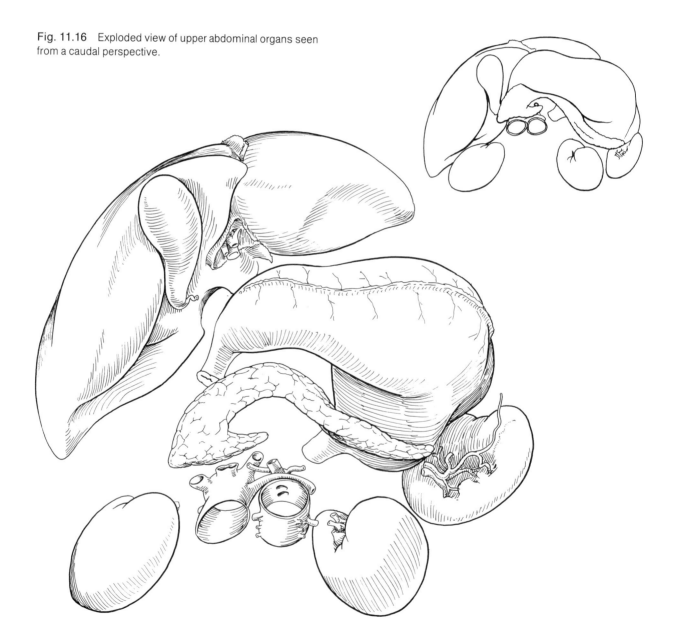

Abdominal Arterial Supply

The major visceral arteries of the abdomen arise close together from the proximal abdominal aorta (Fig. 11.17). Almost immediately after emerging beneath the diaphragmatic crura, the aorta gives rise to the celiac trunk in the midline at about a 90° angle. The superior mesenteric artery arises just distal to the celiac artery and makes a sharply acute angle in the caudal direction. The angles of origin of these two vessels make it more hemodynamically probable for an embolus arising proximally (e.g., a fragment of a cardiac mural thrombus) to enter and occlude the superior mesenteric system and cause bowel ischemia or infarction. The renal arteries arise laterally slightly below the level of the superior mesenteric artery, and the last major midline artery, the inferior mesenteric artery, arises midway between the renal arteries and the aortic bifurcation. Abdominal aortic aneurysms most commonly arise below the level of the renal arteries, and the mural thrombus often occludes the inferior mesenteric artery by the time the aneurysm is discovered and treated. With such gradual occlusion, collateral channels to the inferior mesenteric circulation usually have enlarged enough to prevent compromise of the left colon. Occasionally, when a still patent inferior mesenteric artery is sacrificed during aneurysmectomy and collateral channels are inadequate, ischemia of the left colon may complicate the postoperative course.

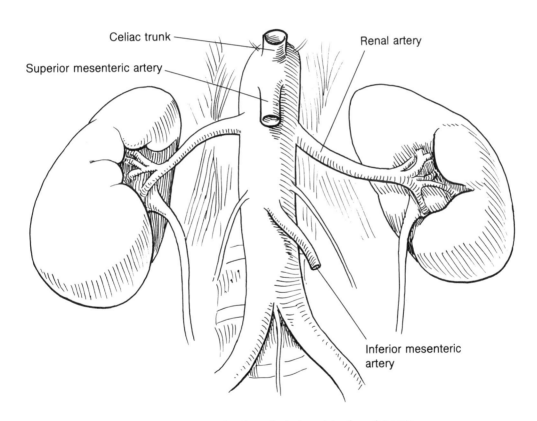

Celiac trunk

Superior mesenteric artery

Renal artery

Inferior mesenteric artery

Fig. 11.17   The major visceral arteries arising from the aorta.

These major arteries roughly divide the abdominal viscera (excluding the pelvis) into four zones (Fig. 11.18). The renal arteries supply the retroperitoneal kidneys and partially supply the adrenals. The celiac artery, with its left gastric, splenic, and hepatic branches, perfuses the upper abdominal organs up to the distal duodenum. The superior mesenteric system supplies the small bowel and the large bowel up to the distal transverse colon. The retroperitoneal pancreas is supplied mainly by branches of the celiac artery, with a small contribution to the pancreatic head by the superior mesenteric artery. The remainder of the colon receives blood from the inferior mesenteric artery and pelvic vessels.

The celiac system richly supplies the stomach with anastomotic loops on both curvatures: left and right gastric arteries along the lesser curve, and left and right gastroepiploic arteries along the greater curve

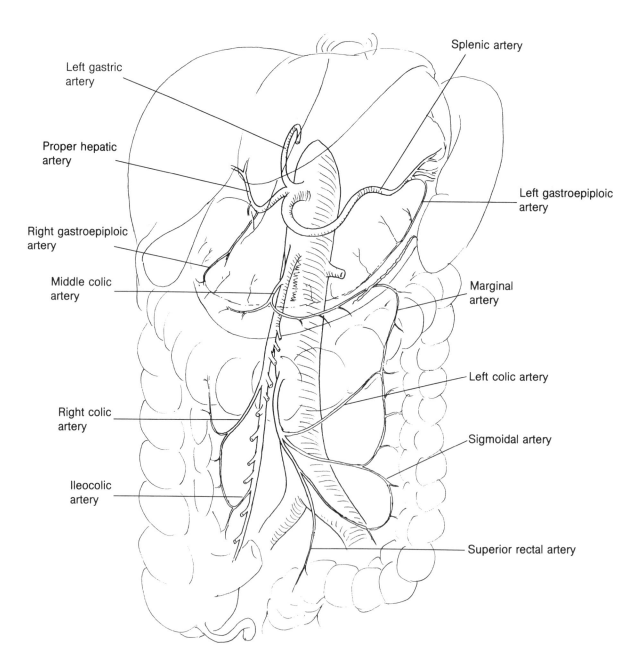

Left gastric artery

Proper hepatic artery

Right gastroepiploic artery

Middle colic artery

Right colic artery

Ileocolic artery

Splenic artery

Left gastroepiploic artery

Marginal artery

Left colic artery

Sigmoidal artery

Superior rectal artery

Fig. 11.18   The distribution of visceral arteries.

(Fig. 11.19). The right gastroepiploic artery arises from the gastroduodenal branch of the common hepatic artery, and the left gastroepiploic artery arises from a terminal branch of the splenic artery. This network can support the stomach even if only one of the four feeding vessels is left intact and allows all or part of the stomach to be mobilized into the chest as a substitute for the esophagus.

The splenic flexure of the colon has a potentially weak blood supply if the arcades connecting the left colic artery and the left branch of the middle colic artery are poorly developed. Thus this area is a poor choice for an anastomotic site after colon resection. When this connecting arcade is large or hypertrophied secondary to inferior mesenteric artery occlusion, it is given the eponym "marginal artery of Drummond."

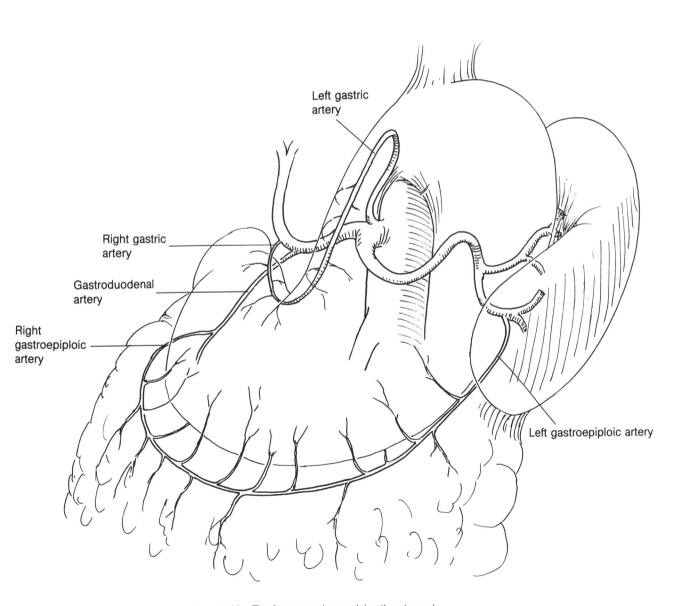

Left gastric artery

Right gastric artery

Gastroduodenal artery

Right gastroepiploic artery

Left gastroepiploic artery

Fig. **11.19** The four vessels supplying the stomach.

Abdominal Venous Drainage

The veins draining the abdominal organs become confluent in the portal vein, which enters the hilum of the liver (Fig. 11.20). After percolating through the hepatic sinusoids, the blood reenters the systemic circulation via the hepatic veins at the posterior rim of the liver dome. The superior mesenteric and splenic veins are the two main channels that unite posterior to the neck of the pancreas to form the portal vein. The inferior mesenteric vein, draining the territory of the inferior mesenteric artery, usually enters the splenic vein behind the body of the pancreas, but may also join the superior mesenteric vein or the superior mesenteric-splenic junction. Smaller tributaries include the pancreatoduodenal veins and the left gastric vein draining the lesser curvature of the stomach. The latter may form a complete circuit with the right gastric vein (Figs. 11.20 and 11.21). After receiving branches from the lower esophagus, the left gastric vein passes through the peritoneal fold containing the left gastric artery and then crosses dorsal to the posterior peritoneum of the omental bursa to reach the portal vein.

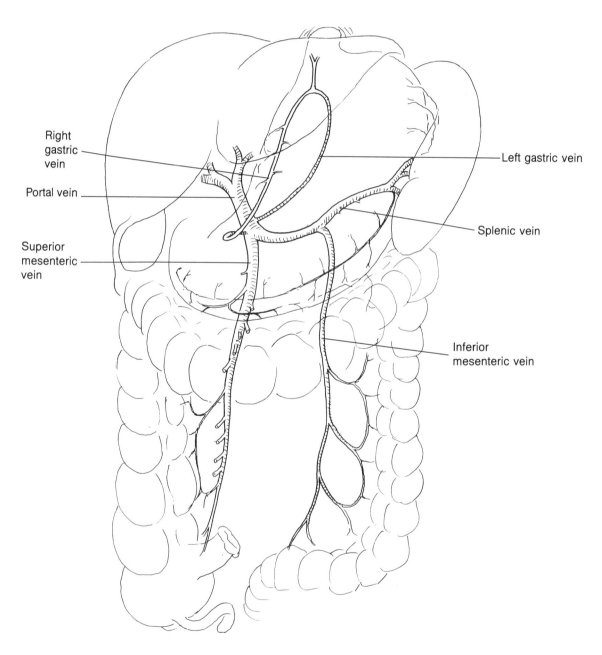

Right gastric vein

Portal vein

Superior mesenteric vein

Left gastric vein

Splenic vein

Inferior mesenteric vein

Fig. 11.20   The hepatic portal system of veins.

When the liver architecture becomes deranged by disease and impedes portal flow, the increased pressure in the portal system is transmitted to peripheral junctures, with potentially serious consequences. The superior rectal branch of the inferior mesenteric vein can cause hemorrhoidal enlargement; the umbilical vein can recanalize, causing periumbilical varices; and the spleen can become enlarged. The most critical varices, however, are those that develop in the lower esophagus as a result of communications to the left gastric vein and to the most cephalad short gastric veins. The submucosal esophageal varices can be eroded by the passage of food and bleed massively. In emergency or intractable situations, the portal system may be decompressed into the systemic circulation by anastomosing the splenic to the left renal vein, the superior mesenteric vein to the inferior vena cava, or the portal vein to the inferior vena cava. The pairs of veins for each of these shunts are in close proximity.

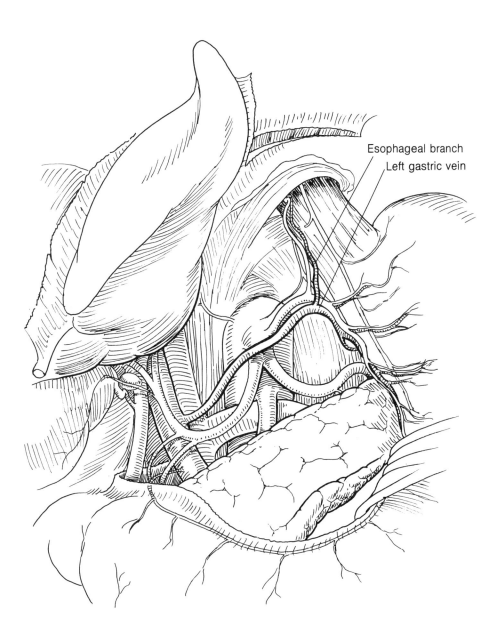

Esophageal branch
Left gastric vein

Fig. 11.21   Relationships of the left gastric vein.

Splenic Relationships

The spleen most commonly requires surgical attention because of blunt abdominal trauma. A knowledge of its architecture and attachments has become more important in recent years with the recognition of the spleen's defensive role in preventing overwhelming sepsis, particularly from pneumococcus. Surgeons now attempt to preserve part or all of the spleen if possible.

The tortuous hilar vessels of the spleen are enfolded by leaves of peritoneum that attach the spleen to surrounding structures (Fig. 11.22). Dorsally the spleen is connected to the fascia overlying the left kidney and to the diaphragm cephalad to the kidney. Anteriorly the main splenic vessels are covered by the peritoneum lining the omental bursa. This layer continues anteriorly and is joined by the reflection of the anterior visceral peritoneum of the spleen to form the gastrosplenic ligament. Sandwiched between the low layers are the gastrosplenic vessels.

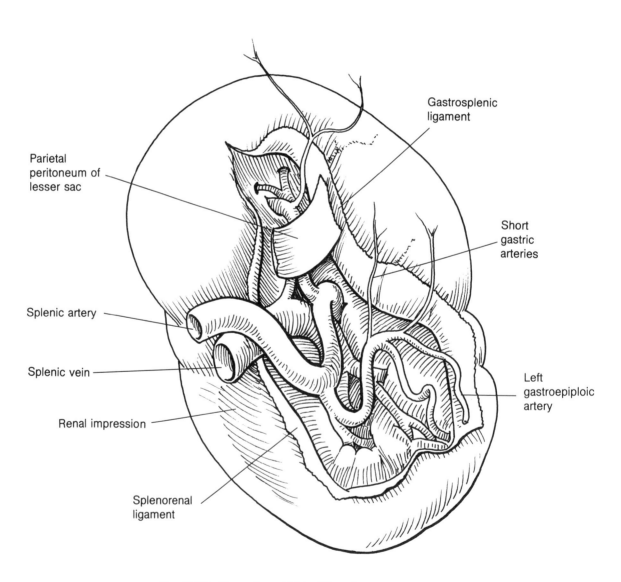

Fig. 11.22   The peritoneal folds of the spleen.

The splenic artery ramifies into several branches before penetrating the splenic substance (Fig. 11.23). Each of these branches supplies a discrete segment of the spleen without significant interconnections. This fact allows segmental resection of the spleen with control of the cut surface by delicate suture of the splenic capsule and topical hemostatic agents.

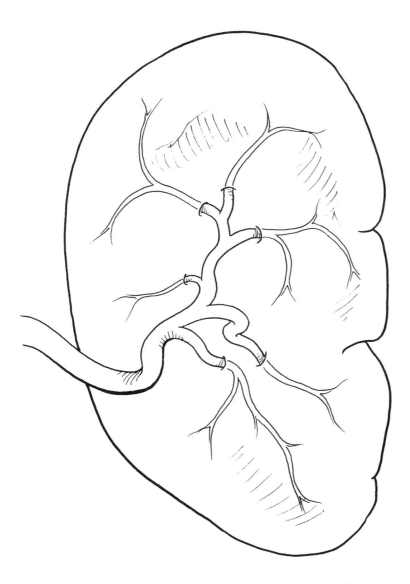

Fig. 11.23   The independent segmental distribution of the terminal splenic artery branches.

Total splenectomy is occasionally required for massive disruption or because of hematological disease. The spleen is situated in the deepest recess of the left subdiaphragmatic space. Good exposure requires considerable retraction of the lower rib cage, regardless of the incision used. The intimate relationship of the spleen to the tail of the pancreas and the splenic flexure of the colon must be kept in mind as mobilization proceeds (Fig. 11.24). The splenic hilum

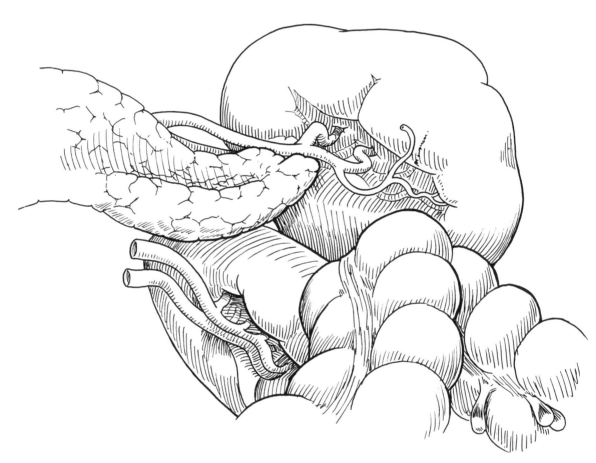

Fig. 11.24   Relationships of the spleen.

is most commonly approached first by dividing the gastrosplenic ligament and working toward the superior pole of the spleen (Fig. 11.25). The short gastric vessels must be securely ligated and even suture ligated to prevent dislodgment of the ligature by postoperative gastric distension. Some surgeons

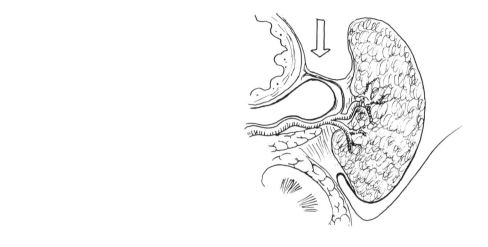

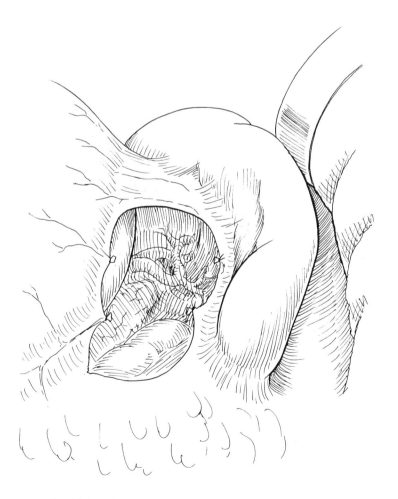

Fig. 11.25   The gastrosplenic ligament.

leave a nasogastric tube in longer after splenectomy than after other abdominal operations to avoid this complication, especially since the operative gastric manipulation and the raw splenic bed predispose to gastric atony. Next the splenorenal ligament is divided (Fig. 11.26), the renal surface of the spleen is gently peeled off the prerenal fascia, and the spleen is elevated to the level of the abdominal wall to expose the hilar vessels either anteriorly or posteriorly. The vessels can then be carefully ligated and suture ligated without injuring the exposed tail of the pancreas.

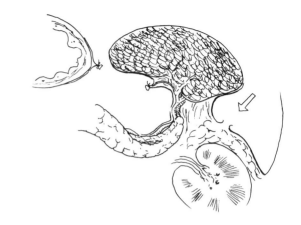

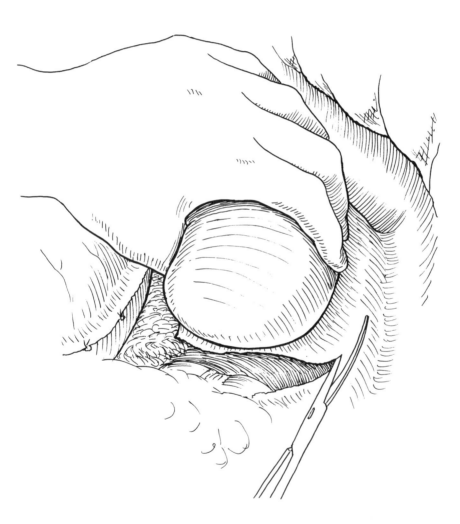

Fig. 11.26   The splenorenal ligament.

Right Upper Quadrant

In an exploded view of the right upper quadrant (Fig. 11.27), one sees several surgically important relationships. Most of the space beneath the right hemidiaphragm is occupied by the volume of the liver. The rim of the costophrenic sulcus interposes pleura between the upper portion of the liver and the lower rib cage. If too deep a puncture is made in performing pleurocentesis for a sympathetic effusion secondary to subphrenic abscess, the abscess may be entered and the pus may infect the pleural fluid, resulting in empyema. A trauma victim with a hemoperitoneum and right lower rib fractures most likely has a liver laceration. Massive injury to the dome of the liver, particularly at the confluence of hepatic veins and vena cava, requires rapid, wide exposure. This is accomplished by a thoracoabdominal incision extending through the lower sternum or into the sixth or seventh intercostal space. Detailed hepatic anatomy is beyond the scope of this discussion, but it should be noted that the division between right and left lobes lies in the plane of the gallbladder fossa and inferior vena cava, not at the falciform ligament. The proximity of the portal structures to the midline should also be noted, as well as the oblique relationship between the portal vein and inferior vena cava. These last two structures lie in the anterior and posterior boundaries of the foramen of Winslow.

The right kidney, adrenal, duodenum, and hepatic flexure of the colon are seated inferior to the right lobe of the liver. The last two structures are often densely adherent after chronic cholecystitis and after prior exploration. Careful dissection is required to avoid injury to the colon, duodenum, and liver. Note the root of the transverse mesocolon overlying the duodenum and the head of the pancreas.

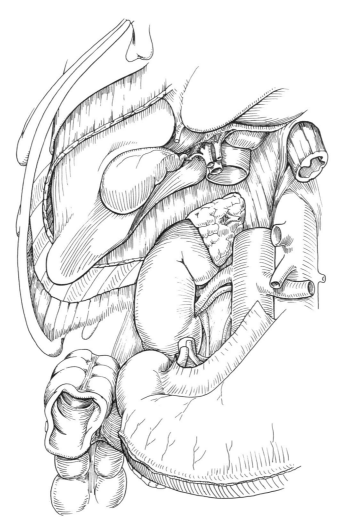

Fig. 11.27 Exploded view of right upper quadrant structures.

Small and Large Bowel Mesentery

The blood vessels, lymphatics, and nerves of the bowel are contained in mesenteries that originate from the posterior parietal peritoneum (Fig. 11.28).

The small bowel and the transverse and sigmoid colon are suspended from well-developed mesenteries covered by peritoneum on both free surfaces. When the right and left colon settled in position during embryonic life, the side of their mesenteries apposed to the posterior parietal peritoneum fused

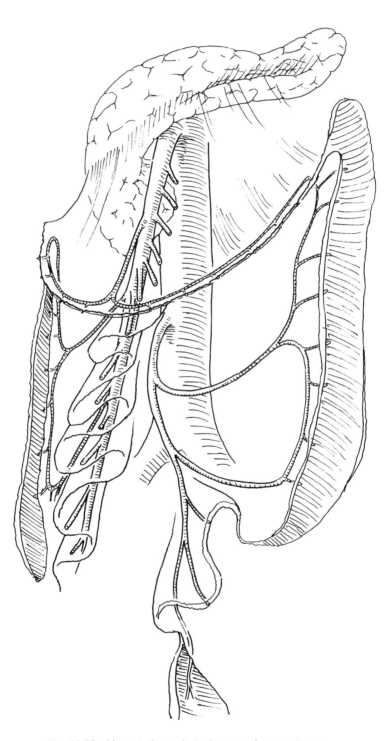

Fig. 11.28 Mesenteries and attachments of the small and large bowel.

with that layer. By gently elevating the right or left colon, the surgeon can make the fusion boundary more prominent and can incise along this so-called white line to mobilize that portion of colon (Fig. 11.29). Staying in the proper avascular plane close to the mesenteric vessels, the surgeon can easily recreate the free mesenteric state of the embryo and expose and protect the underlying ureter and gonadal vessels. In disease states such as diverticulitis, the bowel and mesentery may be bound down to the ureter, and great care must be taken in mobilization.

The root of the small-bowel mesentery traverses the posterior abdominal wall diagonally from upper left to lower right and may direct the diffusion of leaking upper abdominal fluids (e.g., from a perforated duodenal ulcer) toward the right lower quadrant, leading to a mistaken diagnosis of appendicitis. By incising the root of the mesentery to the left of the superior mesenteric artery, the surgeon can expose the abdominal aorta and extend the exposure up to the renal arteries by elevating the duodenum (Fig. 11.30).

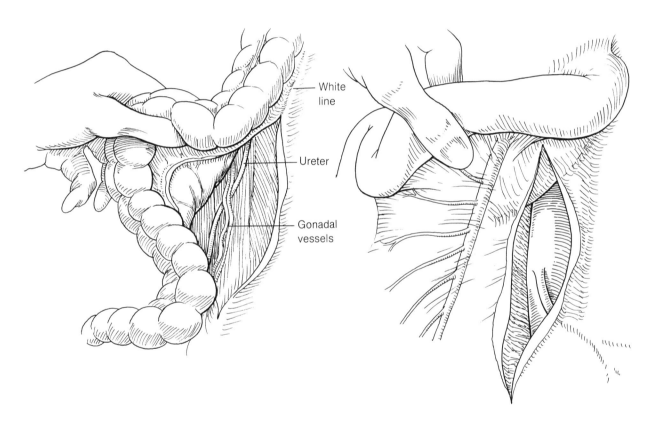

Fig. 11.29 Mobilization of the left colon in the avascular plane.

Fig. 11.30 Opening the root of the small bowel mesentery to expose the infrarenal aorta.

The transverse mesocolon may be quite mobile and may allow the transverse colon to hang low in the abdomen when the patient is upright. Anastomoses between stomach and small bowel can be made in a retrocolic position by opening an avascular part of the transverse mesocolon (Fig. 11.31). The mesocolon is sutured around the stomach to prevent slippage and constriction of the bowel loop by the mobile mesentery. The root of the transverse mesocolon crosses the pancreas and may be involved in pancreatic disease states.

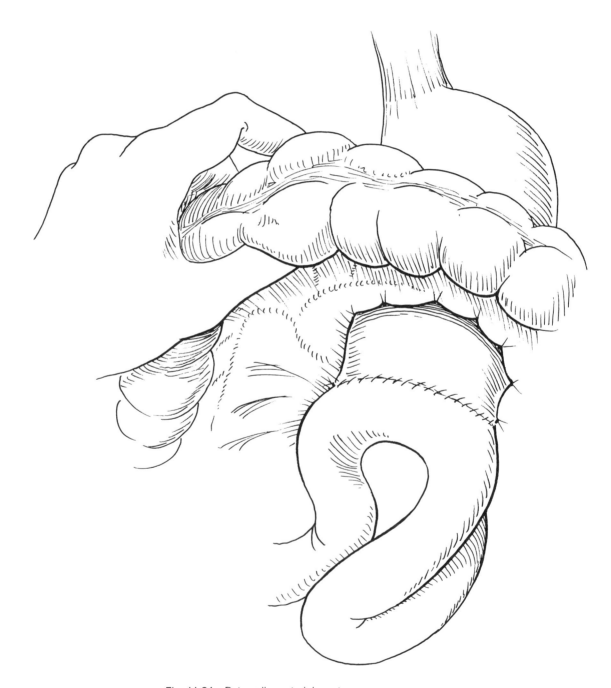

Fig. 11.31   Retrocolic gastrojejunostomy.

Chapter 12

Laparotomy

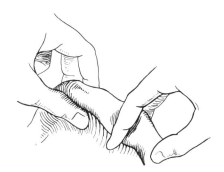

This chapter introduces a series of abdominal operations. Simple general surgical procedures are chosen because they are common to the early training of both general surgeons and surgical specialists. The emphasis is on the principles, which are learned along with these procedures during the formative years of training.

Fine points of surgical technique associated with laparotomy are presented in the following order: opening, freeing adhesions, exploring, closing, and draining the abdomen.

Opening

Prior to the incision, powder is washed off the gloves to reduce the chance of foreign body reaction and consequent intraperitoneal adhesions.

The mechanics of making an incision have been discussed in the chapter on basic surgical maneuvers (Chapter 5). The length, placement, and shape of the incision are as important as technical perfection (Fig. 12.1). Adequate length is necessary to provide exposure for precise anatomical dissection and easy control of serious contingencies. If the incision is long enough, then forceful, traumatic retraction is unnecessary. The operative field is prepared so that anatomical landmarks are evident, and it is draped widely enough so that the incision can be extended easily. The location of the incision is chosen to provide the best exposure within the constraints of the surrounding anatomy. Some incisions must be planned so that they do not limit the surgeon's options for a subsequent procedure (e.g., mastectomy following breast biopsy). The shape of an incision is sometimes dictated by anatomical circumstances (e.g., the areolar margin) and may be modified to follow skin tension lines. A final consideration affecting the incision is cosmetic. An esthetic result is desirable, as long as it does not compromise the effectiveness of the exposure. To leave a patient with an unnecessarily disfiguring scar is contrary to the principle of doing no harm. But to operate through an inadequate incision can result in tragedy – such as common duct injury – far worse than a long scar.

In Fig. 12.2, retraction of subcutaneous tissue upward and outward puts the tissue under maximal tension for a clean incision. The second knife reaches fascia in a few smooth strokes if constant tension is maintained. Hemostasis can then proceed in an orderly fashion as discussed in Chapter 5. The wound may be protected from residual skin bacteria and desiccation with towels or plastic adhesive drapes.

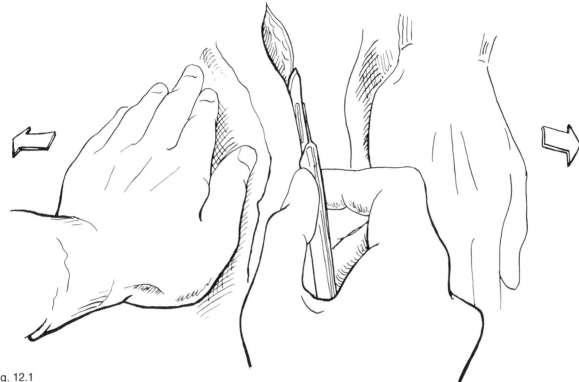

Fig. 12.1

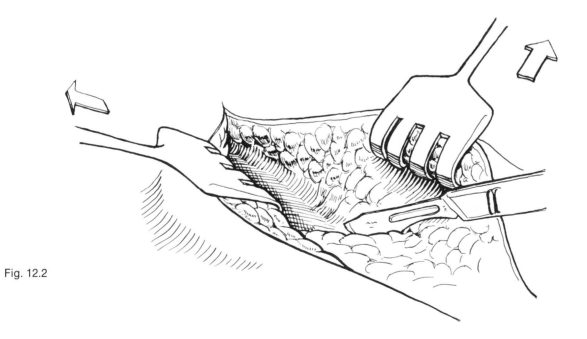

Fig. 12.2

Midline Incision

Tension is maintained on subcutaneous tissue when incising fascia. A gentle stroke with the belly of the blade opens fascia, as in the midline incision shown in Fig. 12.3. As the fascia separates, preperitoneal fat bulges into the incision. The decussation of rectus sheath fibers is a good indicator of midline location.

In Fig. 12.4 a small area of fat is pushed aside with the knife handle to expose the peritoneum. The peritoneum is alternately grasped with forceps by surgeon and assistant until a clear fold containing only peritoneum is tented up. The fold is palpated to make certain no other structure is caught between the layers.

In Fig. 12.5 a small nick is made in the apex of the folds and air is allowed to enter the peritoneal cavity. The incision is best timed to coincide with expiration to allow the abdominal viscera to fall away from the knife blade. Unexpected buckling, especially with distended bowel, can cause a loop of bowel to be impaled on the knife.

The incision is enlarged (Fig. 12.6) to allow insertion of two fingers. Preperitoneal fat is gently pushed aside. Crossing vessels are electrocoagulated or ligated before they are cut or torn. While maintaining tension with his fingers, the surgeon incises the peritoneum in both directions to the full length of the incision.

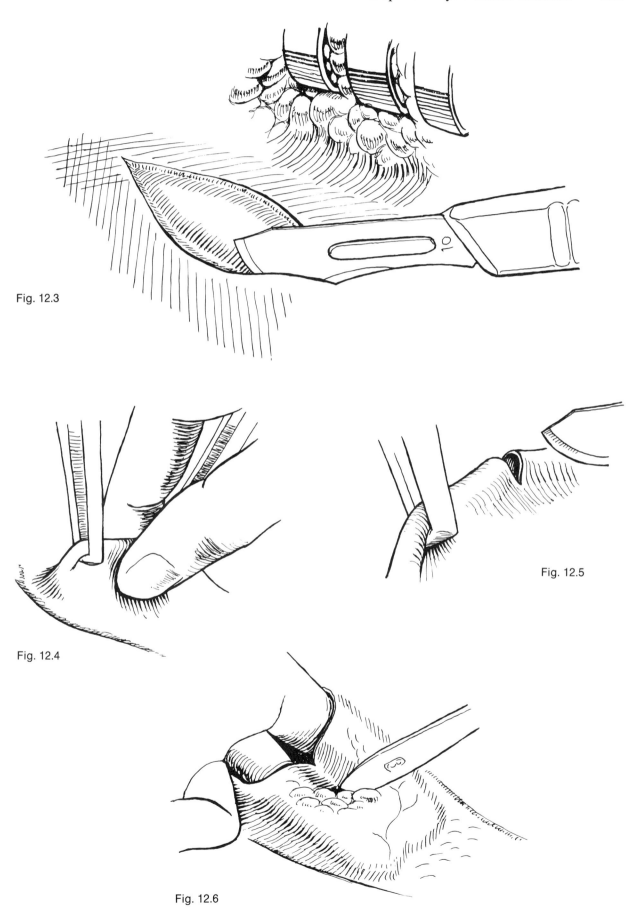

Fig. 12.3

Fig. 12.4

Fig. 12.5

Fig. 12.6

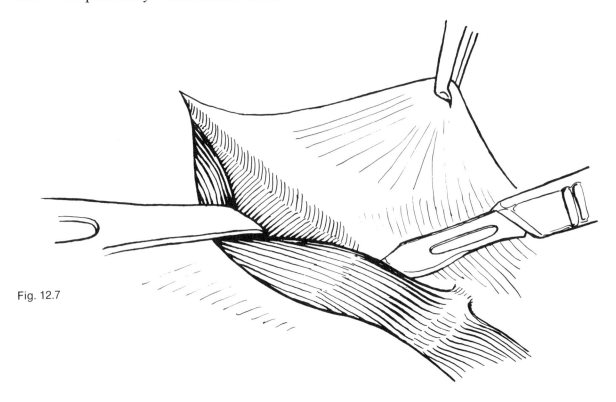

Fig. 12.7

Paramedian Incision

In Fig. 12.7 a paramedian incision opens the anterior rectus sheath. The muscle is then retracted, preferably by sharp dissection. Muscle-splitting incisions are less desirable because the denervated medial strip atrophies.

There is invariably a small blood vessel where the tendinous inscriptions of the rectus muscle attach to the midline fascia (Fig. 12.8). The attachment may be clamped prior to division in some cases, but often a broad attachment dictates cutting across first and controlling the bleeder later.

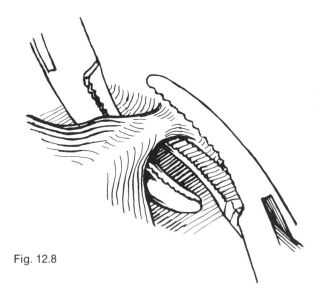

Fig. 12.8

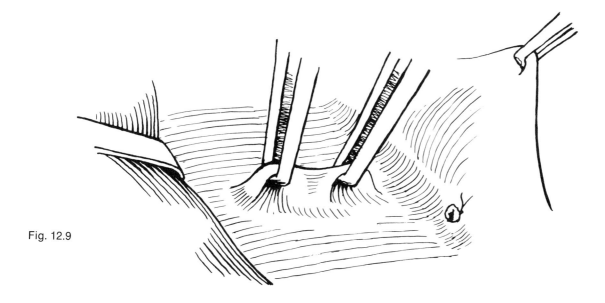

Fig. 12.9

In Fig. 12.9 the posterior rectus sheath and peritoneum are elevated in the same manner as was the peritoneum in the midline incision, and an opening is made.

Discussion of a muscle-splitting incision is found in Chapter 13 (Appendectomy), and of a transverse incision in Chapter 15 (Cholecystectomy).

Adhesions

Adhesions are most often found in a previously operated abdomen. Individuals vary widely in the number of adhesions they form. A fourth laparotomy in one patient may reveal a clear abdomen; a second look in another patient may present a solid wall of adhesions. It is a good practice to use a previous incision and extend it in order to enter the peritoneum in a clean area, since the greatest density of adhesions is likely to be directly under the scar. In Fig. 12.10, once a small opening into the peritoneum is found, it is delicately enlarged to provide a fascial edge that can be grasped and elevated.

In Fig. 12.11 the surgeon's left index finger gently elevates the adhesion between the bowel and parietal peritoneum while the thumb rolls the bowel away, revealing the edge. This retraction and exposure defines the relatively avascular area of adhesion that may be safely incised. Although adhesions constitute abnormal anatomical connections and are divided to recreate normal planes, they may contain numerous fine parasitic vessels, which leave a raw, oozing surface when cut. For this reason lysis of adhesions should be limited to essential areas unless a complete exploration is necessary. All the raw surfaces will again become adherent once the abdomen is closed. The dissection proceeds logically from superficial to deep, bringing the entire field to the same level without creating a deep hole. Gentle sharp dissection prevents serosal avulsion. There is no reason why any secondary laparotomy must be accompanied by multiple accidental enterotomies. Those who excuse such an occurrence on the the basis of difficulty are usually excusing poor technique.

Some adhesions, such as those between loops of bowel, lend themselves to scissors dissection, as shown in Fig. 12.12. Basic principles must be followed – i.e., cut only what can be seen, do not lose sight of the point, do not poke, and open the scissors only enough to define the plane. Manipulation of the bowel is kept to a minimum to prevent prolonged ileus. For additional comments on adhesions, refer to Chapter 15.

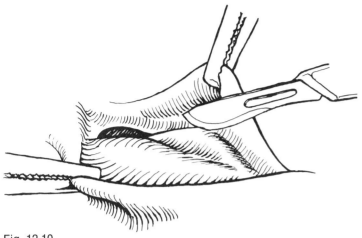

Fig. 12.10

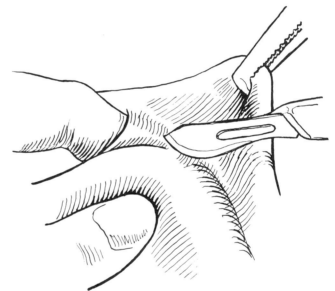

Fig. 12.11

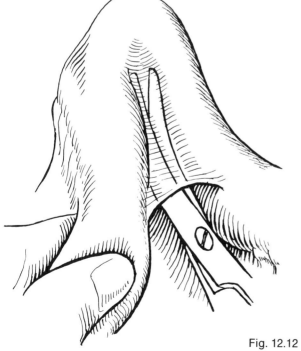

Fig. 12.12

Exploration

In order not to omit any part of a complete exploration, it is helpful to establish a routine pattern. The sequence that follows is one such pattern. It follows the course of the gastrointestinal tract, starting in the upper abdomen, and examines the retroperitoneal organs as they are encountered. Vertical incisions allow the most thorough exploration; other incisions may impose limitations. The lateral segment of the left lobe of the liver is immediately accessible. One hand slides over the cephalad surface up to the left triangular ligament. A second hand is placed under the caudal surface, and bimanual palpation for deep parenchymal lesions is performed. If the round ligament is not divided, the hand must slide under it to palpate the rest of the liver to the right of the falciform ligament (Fig. 12.13). The dome is palpated as far posterior as the suspensory ligaments, and bimanual exam again is performed. This maneuver will allow air to enter between diaphragm and liver, causing the liver to descend into the field. The gallbladder is palpated for stones. The common duct is felt in the edge of the hepatoduodenal ligament. A heavy clamp on the cut end of the round ligament provides excellent traction for hepatic manipulation.

The surgeon now checks the left upper quadrant, keeping the dorsum of the hand pressed up against the parietal peritoneum of the anterior abdominal wall, as shown in Fig. 12.14. He gently examines the spleen for size and consistency, without tearing short gastric vessels. Rough handling of the ligamentous attachments can cause avulsion of the splenic capsule. A rim of the cephalad and lateral portion of the left kidney may be felt posteriorly.

Further steps in exploration are shown and discussed in Fig. 12.15–12.23.

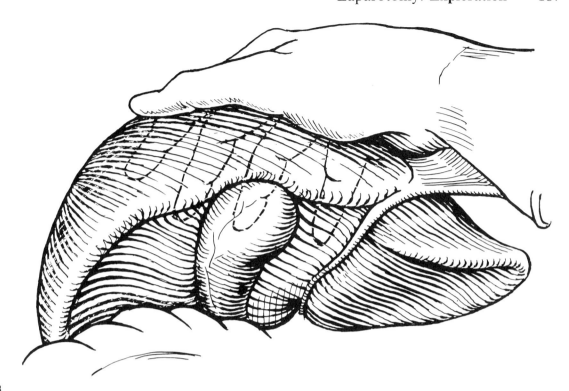

Fig. 12.13

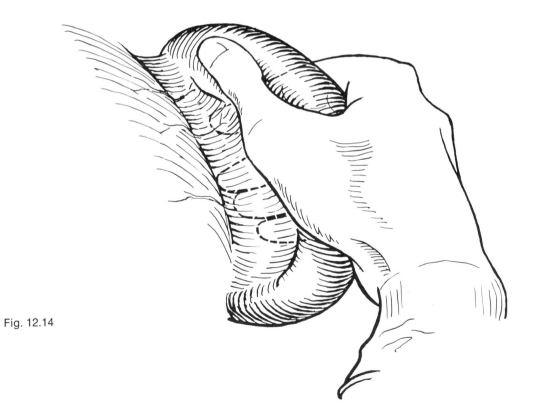

Fig. 12.14

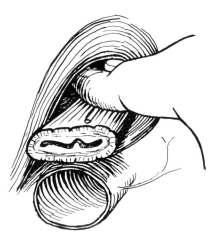

Fig. 12.15   With his hand between liver and proximal stomach, the surgeon identifies the esophageal hiatus by feeling for the pulsation of the underlying aorta. A normal hiatus admits the tips of one to two fingers. For clarity, the overlying peritoneum is omitted from this diagram.

Fig. 12.16   The fundus and body of the stomach are palpated with the flattened hand, keeping in mind the position of the underlying pancreas. Gross abnormalities of the body and tail of the pancreas may be appreciated in this way, but accurate evaluation requires entering the lesser sac through the gastrocolic omentum. The celiac axis area is palpated cephalad to the lesser curve of the stomach. The most common abnormality is lymphadenopathy.

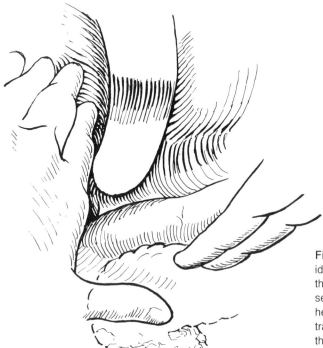

Fig. 12.17   The antrum is examined, and the pylorus is identified by the characteristic pyloric veins. The pylorus and the first portion of the duodenum are examined for scarring secondary to peptic ulcer disease. The exposed portion of the head of the pancreas is palpated through the root of the transverse mesocolon. A thorough examination of the head of the pancreas involves mobilization by the Kocher maneuver (incising the peritoneal attachment of the duodenum and elevating the duodenum and pancreatic head).

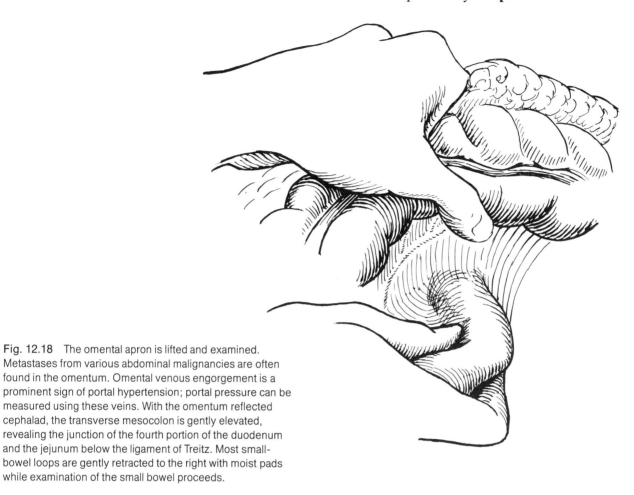

Fig. 12.18   The omental apron is lifted and examined. Metastases from various abdominal malignancies are often found in the omentum. Omental venous engorgement is a prominent sign of portal hypertension; portal pressure can be measured using these veins. With the omentum reflected cephalad, the transverse mesocolon is gently elevated, revealing the junction of the fourth portion of the duodenum and the jejunum below the ligament of Treitz. Most small-bowel loops are gently retracted to the right with moist pads while examination of the small bowel proceeds.

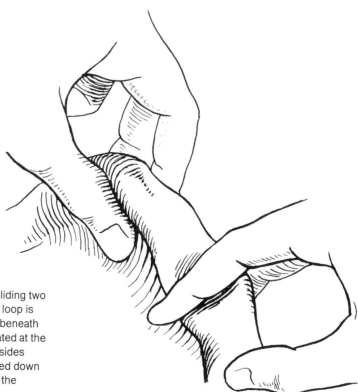

Fig. 12.19   The small bowel is examined by gently sliding two fingers along the loop to feel for polyps. The proximal loop is supported with fingertips apposed on the mesentery beneath the bowel wall. When the hands are maximally separated at the end of each segment, the loop is flipped so that both sides have been directly visualized. The process is continued down to the iliocecal valve. The distal ileum is examined for the presence of a Meckel's diverticulum.

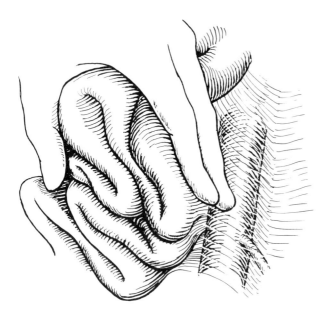

Fig. 12.20   With the small bowel reflected to the right, the aorta may be palpated. The lower pole of the left kidney may be felt to the left of the aorta, beneath the root of the transverse mesocolon.

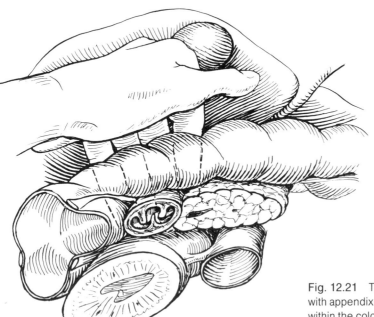

Fig. 12.21   The large bowel is now carefully palpated, starting with appendix and cecum. It is easy to miss small lesions within the colon, and it is difficult to differentiate stool from polyps in an unprepped colon. At the hepatic flexure the hand can slide over the colon and duodenum and beneath the liver to reach Morrison's pouch. There the upper portion of the right kidney can be felt. Morrison's pouch, the most posterior accessible recess of the upper peritoneal cavity, provides excellent access for drainage of a right subphrenic abscess through the bed of the 12th rib immediately posterior to it.

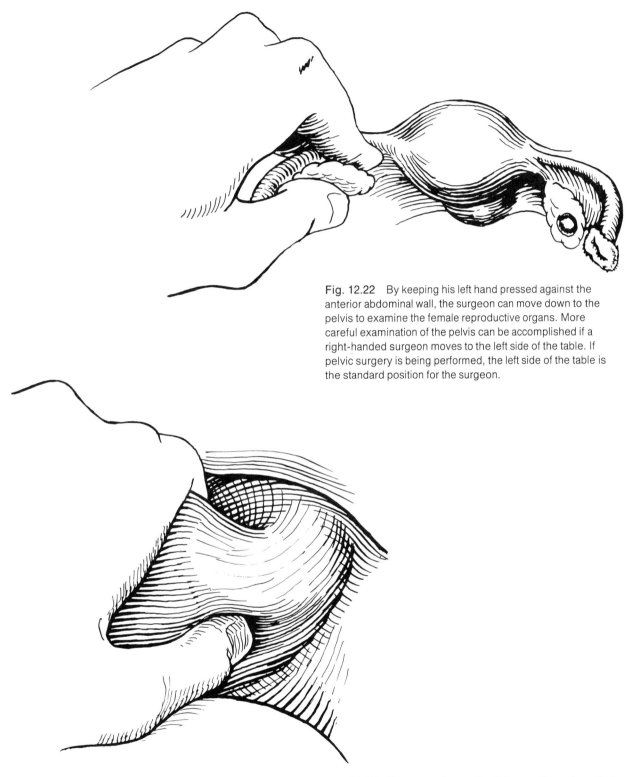

Fig. 12.22 By keeping his left hand pressed against the anterior abdominal wall, the surgeon can move down to the pelvis to examine the female reproductive organs. More careful examination of the pelvis can be accomplished if a right-handed surgeon moves to the left side of the table. If pelvic surgery is being performed, the left side of the table is the standard position for the surgeon.

Fig. 12.23 The rectum is examined down to the rectovaginal or rectovesical recess, the most caudal point in the peritoneal cavity. Pelvic lymph nodes are found along the course of the major vessels. The ureters are best identified where they cross the external iliac vessels.

Closure

The completion of a one-layer, figure-of-eight abdominal closure is depicted in Figures 12.24–12.26. Paramedian and transverse incisions may lend themselves more easily to a multilayer technique. The important principle illustrated here holds true for any type of closure: the sutures that complete peritoneal closure must be placed and tightened with exquisite care to avoid catching bowel. In Fig. 12.24 the last three sutures have been placed but not tightened. A finger is inserted in one direction to ensure that the incision and sutures at that end are free from underlying structures.

In Fig. 12.25, while the assistant holds snug the two previously examined sutures, the surgeon sweeps his finger around to check the other end of the incision.

The surgeon then slowly removes his finger as he keeps tension on the final suture (Fig. 12.26). Each suture is tied in turn while tension is maintained on the others. Putting in the last few sutures without tying also allows adherence to the principle of working under direct vision.

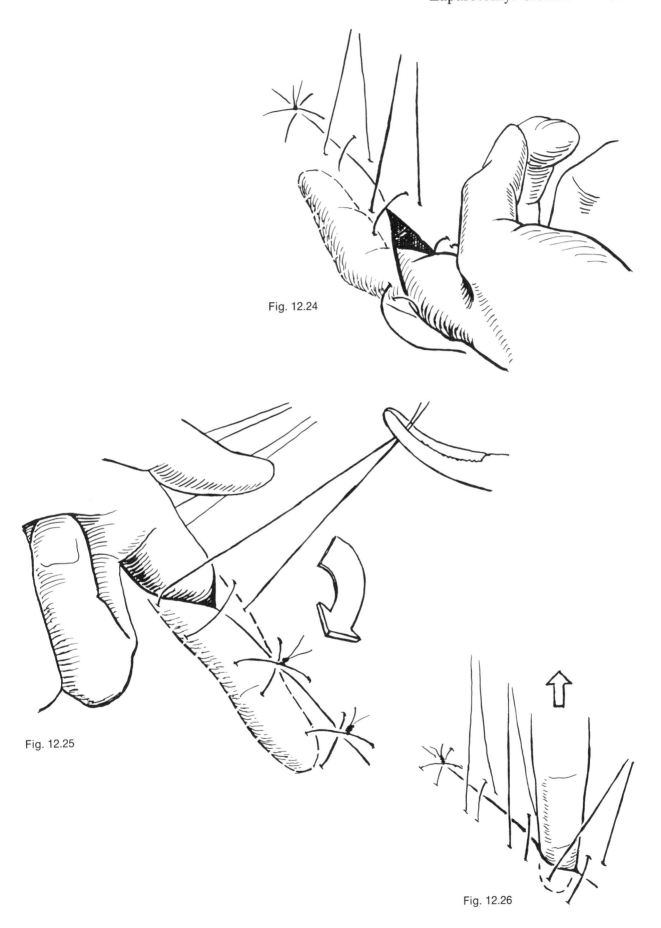

Fig. 12.24

Fig. 12.25

Fig. 12.26

Retention Sutures

Retention sutures are large-diameter (Nos. 1–5) sutures passed through the full thickness of the abdominal wall; they are used to help close the abdomen in special circumstances. Since they allow a rapid closure, they can be used alone in mass casualty situations. In more elective circumstances they can supplement the standard abdominal closure. As the name implies, they may be left in for long periods to guard against wound dehiscence in high-risk situations such as massive trauma, gross contamination, intestinal obstruction (where there is a risk of prolonged postoperative ileus and distension), patients on high-dose steroids, chronically debilitated patients (cancer, inflammatory bowel disease), patients with ascites, and the elderly and obese.

Retention sutures come on long curved cutting needles, which are held close to the suture end for maximum penetration. In Fig. 12.27 the surgeon's left hand is cupped between the needle and viscera as the needle is passed through the abdominal wall. On the side opposite, the surgeon passes the needle backhand, again protecting the viscera and elevating the abdominal wall with the left hand. In this illustration all layers (including peritoneum) are included in the stitch. If the stitches are placed in this way, one must be extra careful not to trap bowel as the suture is tightened. Until they are tied, the sutures may be carefully drawn up and clamped at skin level to maintain tension.

The retention suture may also be placed extraperitoneally (that is, through all layers but peritoneum). This provides some extra security against trapping bowel and helps protect the underlying bowel from the sawing effect of direct contact with the suture. The suture should be tied just snugly enough to admit two fingertips, as shown in Fig. 12.28. This compensates for postoperative wound edema and prevents the suture from cutting through tissue by pressure necrosis. A variety of bridges is available to help prevent the sutures from cutting. Simple rubber tubing is shown here.

When retention sutures are used in high-risk situations, the skin should be left open with packing between the sutures to decrease the chance of infection. The fascia may be closed as shown in Fig. 12.29, and the retention sutures can be used as an adjunct. With the retention sutures not bearing all the tension, they are less likely to cut through. Wound dehiscence usually results from infection and fascial necrosis. When a gap in the fascia develops, the underlying bowel pushes up against the bridging retention sutures, and pressure necrosis of the bowel wall leads to fistula formation. This sequence of events can occur under a closed skin surface. Thus, for the sake of monitoring as well as prophylaxis against infection, it is wisest to leave such high-risk wounds open.

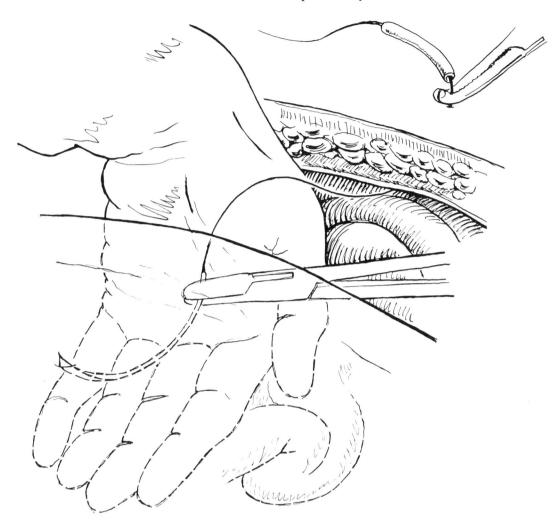

Fig. 12.27

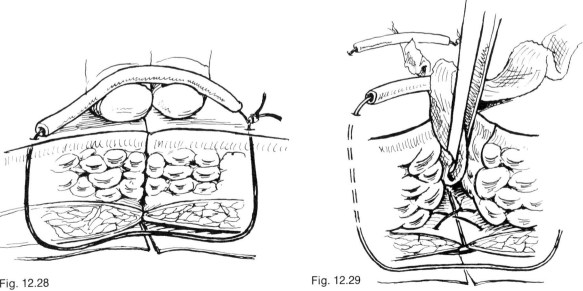

Fig. 12.28

Fig. 12.29

Abdominal and Soft Tissue Drains

Fluid collection at an operative site is often a natural consequence of surgery, and pathological fluid collections such as abscesses often require drainage. It is therefore necessary for the surgeon to be familiar with the principles of surgical drainage and the types of drainage devices available. These principles concern the risks, indications, contraindications, placement, and removal of drains, and they are the subject of this section. The discussion here focuses on abdominal drainage, but the principles apply to all areas.

Historical Perspective

Historically, woven materials such as linen and rigid materials such as Hippocrates' tin tube were used for tissue drainage. Up to the 19th century, abdominal drainage was done only for the relief of ascites. When Ephraim McDowell successfully removed a large diseased ovary in 1809, other surgeons were emboldened to operate in the abdomen. These surgeons observed abdominal fluid collections in patients who died after surgery (5 of McDowell's 13 patients died) and associated these collections with the cause of death. Their expectation that such collections could be drained transvaginally was based on the historical experience with freely draining ascites but was frustrated by the rapid walling off of drains placed in the peritoneal cavity. Faced with these failures of drainage, Mikulicz in 1881 emphasized the importance of eliminating dead space to prevent fluid collection, and surgeons began to reclose the peritoneum over raw surfaces. In the last quarter of the 19th century, the role of infectious agents colonizing the fluid collection was recognized, and aseptic techniques were developed. Despite progress in surgical technique and aseptic practices, the need for drainage persisted, as did the problems. A remarkable variety of materials were tried, including decalcified bone, animal arteries, horsehair, wool, silk, catgut, asbestos, glass, gauze, and rubber.

In the late 19th century, attempts were made to overcome the problems inherent in the drainage practices of the time. Gauze drains, which theoretically worked by capillary action, were subject to tissue ingrowth and adherence; they had to be removed after 2–3 days and be replaced by tubes made of hard rubber or perforated glass. In 1882 Kehrer was the first to enclose gauze in a nonporous sheath, which was made of firm rubber. In 1897 Penrose described a new drain consisting of gauze enclosed in a soft rubber sheath made by cutting the end off a condom. The Penrose drain is still widely used for passive drainage but without the gauze wick (Fig. 12.30). In most applications today active suction drains of the sump or closed type have largely supplanted open passive drainage.

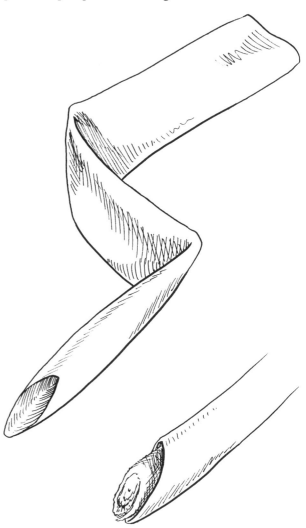

Fig. 12.30   The Penrose is the most commonly used soft rubber drain.

Risks

Surgical drains cannot compensate for sloppy surgery and carry risks of their own. The open drain provides a channel for possible entry of bacteria and may act as a foreign body that harbors bacteria. For this reason drains are seldom used in joint spaces or near prosthetic vascular grafts, or brought directly out through a surgical incision. Drains, especially those made of hard material, may cause pressure necrosis of soft tissue and lead to fecal fistulae and erosion of blood vessels. A drain itself may act as an irritant and stimulate persistent low-grade drainage, a factor that must be considered when choosing the time to remove a drain. A opening made in the body wall for the drain to exit may become a site of future weakness and hernia. For all these reasons the choice, placement, and care of drains must be cautious and appropriate. The advent of soft synthetic materials and closed drainage devices has made these tasks easier in the past several years.

Indications and Contraindications

Surgical drains (excluding gastrointestinal drainage tubes and bladder catheters) are indicated for therapeutic and prophylactic evacuation of fluid accumulations in the body. Most therapeutic drainage is done for infected fluid that may be walled off (abscess), generalized (e.g., peritonitis), or contained in a ductal system in the case of cholangitis. Walled-off abscesses are essentially treated by the act of drainage,

but the inflammatory process that walled off the infection often leaves stiff walls that will not collapse to obliterate the space. The purpose of a drain in this case is to keep the opening (which must be adequately large to start with) patent while the cavity gradually closes and to prevent reformation of the abscess. A Penrose and/or firm rubber tube (Fig. 12.31) is sufficient for this purpose. Generalized peritonitis is primarily treated by laparotomy, surgical correction of the initiating pathology, and antibiotics. After such a laparotomy, some surgeons will drain the abdomen with large sump drains (Fig. 12.32) in the hope of preventing subsequent abscesses or giving an abscess a formed tract to break into and drain through. Because the drain tract becomes walled off in 24–48 hours, other surgeons feel that this is a futile practice and rely on the antibiotics alone. The drains can also be used for irrigation and antibiotic instillation, at least initially. Acute suppurative cholangitis may require surgical intervention and placement of a T-tube that is attached to straight gravity drainage.

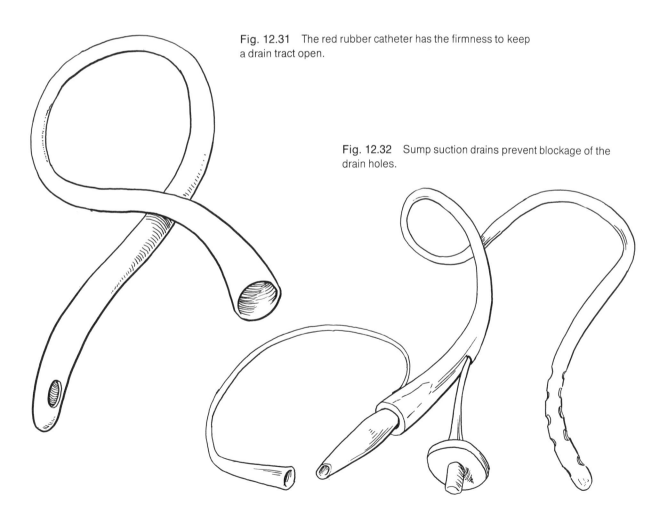

Fig. 12.31   The red rubber catheter has the firmness to keep a drain tract open.

Fig. 12.32   Sump suction drains prevent blockage of the drain holes.

When significant fluid accumulation is a risk after surgery, drains are placed prophylactically. A critical example of this indication is after thyroid surgery when an expanding hematoma could compress the trachea. In other less critical situations (e.g., after mastectomy, colon resection, pelvic surgery) when large raw surfaces are prone to weep fluid, elective drainage decreases the likelihood of such culture media fostering bacterial growth. Closed suction drains are very effective in that situation (Fig. 12.33). The large skin flaps of a mastectomy sometimes continue to ooze after the drain tubing has become occluded with fibrin. In that case the drain tubing is removed, and sterile needle aspiration of accumulated fluid is performed as necessary until the flaps adhere. In many cases the decision whether or not to drain is not clear cut and must be based on the surgeon's judgment and experience. Draining the gallbladder bed after cholecystectomy is one such choice; there has been a trend over the past several years to not drain.

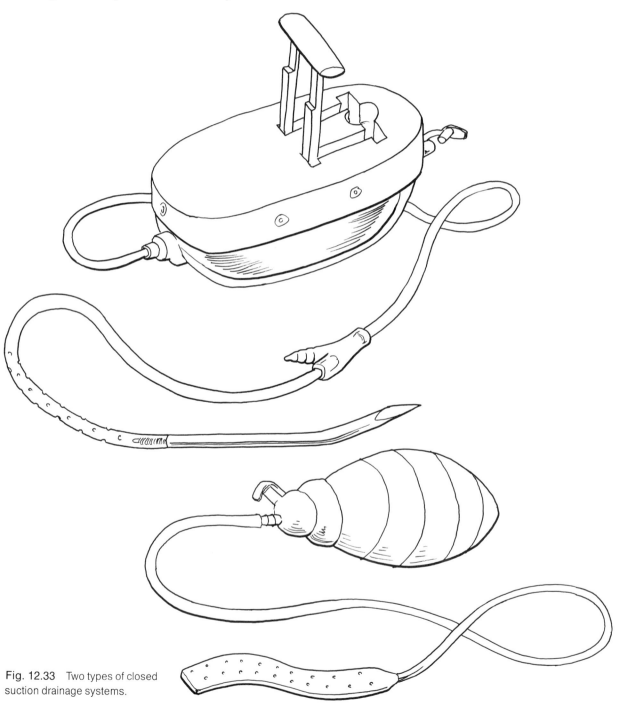

Fig. 12.33 Two types of closed suction drainage systems.

Placement

The placement of drains follows several straightforward guidelines. Drains should reach the skin by the shortest, most direct route. This is particularly important with the large-stemmed T-tubes, which were introduced after the advent of percutaneous residual stone retrieval using the Dormia basket. Such manipulation is facilitated by the straight tract. The stab wound for a drain should be separate from the main incision to prevent soilage and should be just large enough for the drain to pass without constriction. Drains should be placed in dependent recesses where fluid and debris accumulate – for example, the space between the liver and the kidney on the right (see Fig. 11.9), or the space between the rectum and bladder or the rectum and vagina (see Fig. 11.15) – and away from anastomoses, blood vessels, and nerves. Soft drains should be transfixed with a safety pin to prevent them from slipping into the cavity they are draining. All drains should be sutured to skin initially, and tubular drains must be securely taped in such a way that the tape can be easily removed without pulling the drain (Fig. 12.34). Drains should always be handled with sterile technique.

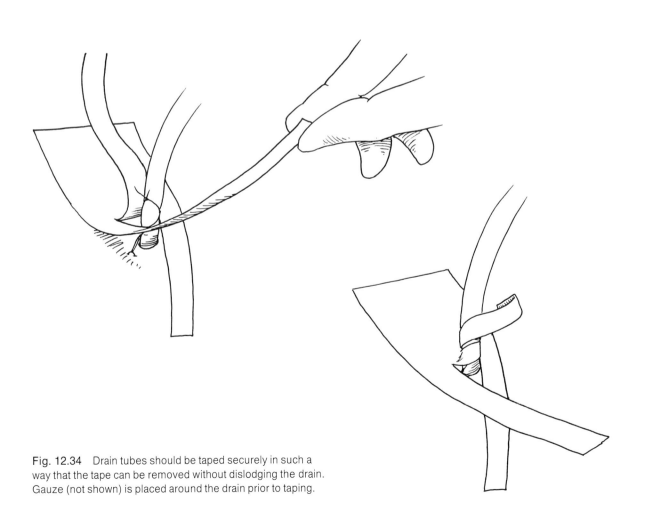

Fig. 12.34   Drain tubes should be taped securely in such a way that the tape can be removed without dislodging the drain. Gauze (not shown) is placed around the drain prior to taping.

Removal

The removal of drains is based on the type of drain and the amount of drainage. Passive drains such as the Penrose will usually drain significantly for the first 24–48 hours until accumulated fluid is evacuated and the drain tract becomes walled off by fibrin. Withdrawing the drain a short distance each subsequent day allows the residual cavity to close from the bottom up and may break up the fibrinous tract, allowing loculations to drain. After the drain is moved, the safety pin is replaced at its new position near the skin, and the excess drain is cut off to decrease the risk of contamination. If drainage persists after this type of drain is removed, the Penrose may be replaced with a straight red rubber catheter. Sump drains are removed when drainage becomes negligible and must be totally withdrawn the first time they are moved since they will not function with some holes in and some out of the cavity. These are usually placed alongside Penrose drains, and the latter are then sequentially withdrawn. Closed suction drains are removed when drainage is no longer significant, which usually occurs before the tubing becomes obstructed. Decreasing drainage from a T-tube indicates that edema of the ampulla secondary to surgical manipulation is subsiding and that a residual stone is not blocking the distal duct. If the T-tube cholangiogram proves normal, the T-tube is pulled after a 24-hour interval to ensure that there is no cholangitis resulting from the cholangiogram. The tract rapidly closes since the bile finds less resistance through the normal physiological channel.

Drain manipulations must be recorded in the patient's chart so that all persons caring for the patient are aware of the current status. For example, it is not uncommon for a slight bacteremia and fever spike to follow drain manipulation, and the record will help pinpoint the cause.

Chapter 13

Appendectomy

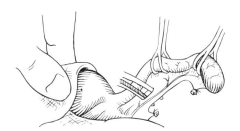

This chapter depicts an operation for acute appendicitis. Surgery is performed as soon as possible after diagnosis to prevent rupture, especially in children and the elderly. Deaths caused by appendicitis are due to complications following rupture. It is far easier to prevent complications than to treat them. Preoperative resuscitation is based on the patient's clinical state.

Fig. 13.1 The McBurney incision is depicted here. It crosses a point two thirds of the distance from umbilicus to right anterior superior spine of ilium. In many patients this location is too close to the lateral border of the rectus sheath, and a slight lateral shift is helpful. The appendix is variable in position; the point of maximum tenderness helps the surgeon place his incision properly. A transverse skin incision is a popular alternative. The incision is made large enough (e.g., 4 cm in an adult) to provide for good exposure for an "easy" appendectomy. It can then be enlarged or extended if difficulty is encountered. It can easily be closed if unexpected findings necessitate a major laparotomy. When the history and physical examination favor a diagnosis of appendicitis, it is logical to start with the least invasive incision.

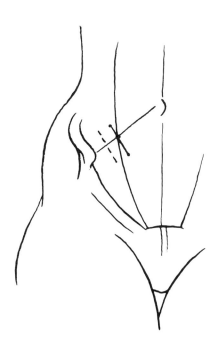

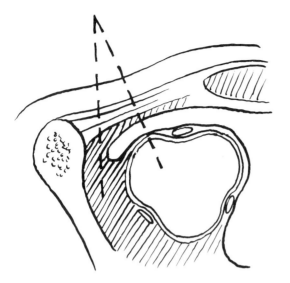

Fig. 13.2   The incision is directed perpendicular to the peritoneum, which curves to follow the iliac bone. Proceeding vertically toward the table top, it is possible to miss the peritoneum entirely. Entry into this retroperitoneal plane is desirable when draining an appendiceal abscess but is not desirable when removing an acutely inflamed appendix.

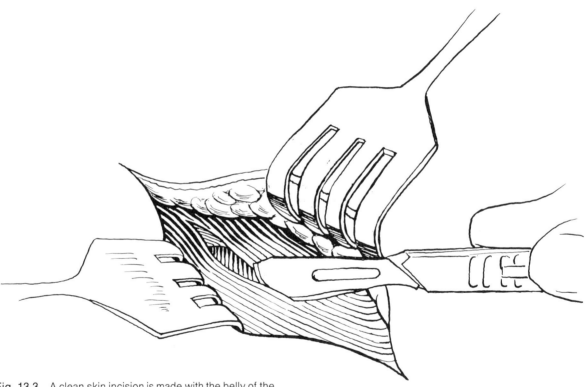

Fig. 13.3   A clean skin incision is made with the belly of the blade. The second knife incises subcutaneous tissue down to the external oblique fascia. Each layer is incised the full length of the incision. Significant bleeders are controlled at this time, as previously described. Small points of subcutaneous ooze will stop. The area is again checked for hemostasis prior to closure. Limiting use of electrocoagulation minimizes trauma. The external oblique layer is opened in the line of its fibers from the muscular portion to the edge of the rectus sheath. Avoid undermining and stripping the fine vessels on the fascial surface. Devascularizing fascia predisposes to necrosis and infection.

Pads or towels cover skin up to the edges of the incision.

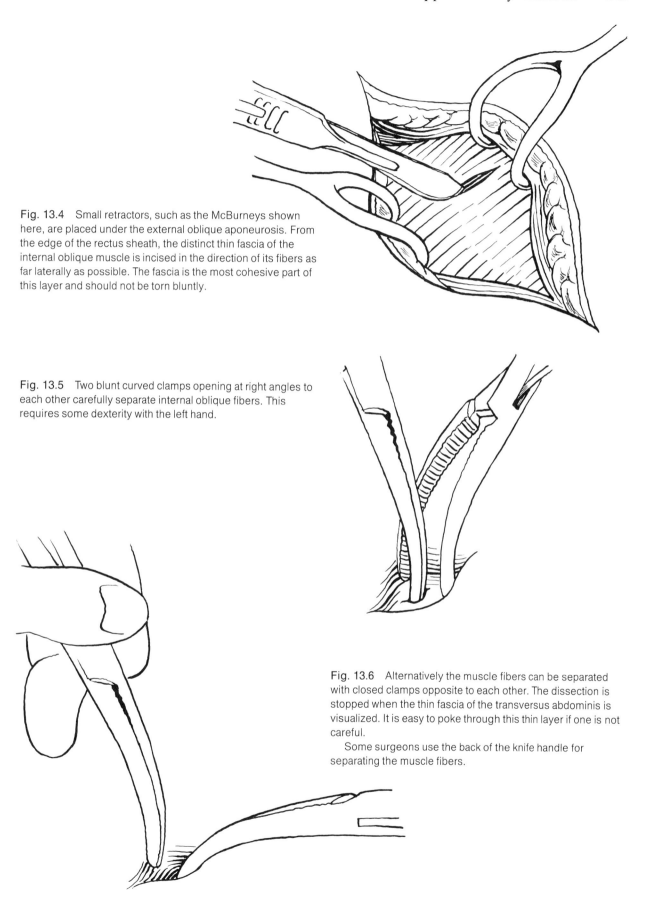

Fig. 13.4   Small retractors, such as the McBurneys shown here, are placed under the external oblique aponeurosis. From the edge of the rectus sheath, the distinct thin fascia of the internal oblique muscle is incised in the direction of its fibers as far laterally as possible. The fascia is the most cohesive part of this layer and should not be torn bluntly.

Fig. 13.5   Two blunt curved clamps opening at right angles to each other carefully separate internal oblique fibers. This requires some dexterity with the left hand.

Fig. 13.6   Alternatively the muscle fibers can be separated with closed clamps opposite to each other. The dissection is stopped when the thin fascia of the transversus abdominis is visualized. It is easy to poke through this thin layer if one is not careful.

Some surgeons use the back of the knife handle for separating the muscle fibers.

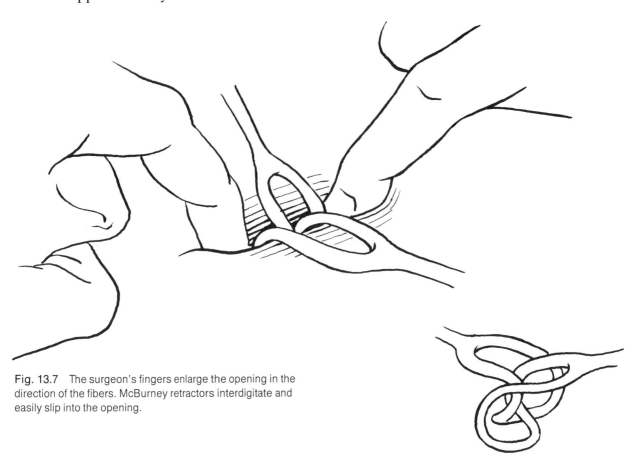

Fig. 13.7 The surgeon's fingers enlarge the opening in the direction of the fibers. McBurney retractors interdigitate and easily slip into the opening.

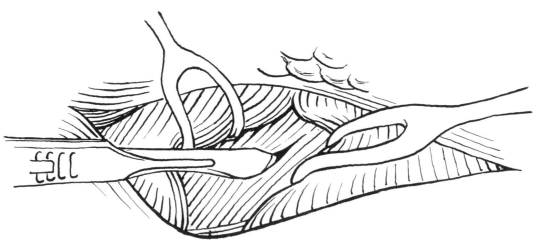

Fig. 13.8 Care should be taken to avoid tissue trauma when retracting the internal oblique muscle. In addition, the iliohypogastric nerve and its associated vessels lie laterally between internal oblique and transversus muscles. Excessive traction will tear the vessels and endanger the nerve.

The fascia of the internal oblique muscle is incised, and muscle fibers are separated as before. The transversus muscle is thinner than the internal oblique, and care should be taken not to enter the peritoneum prematurely.

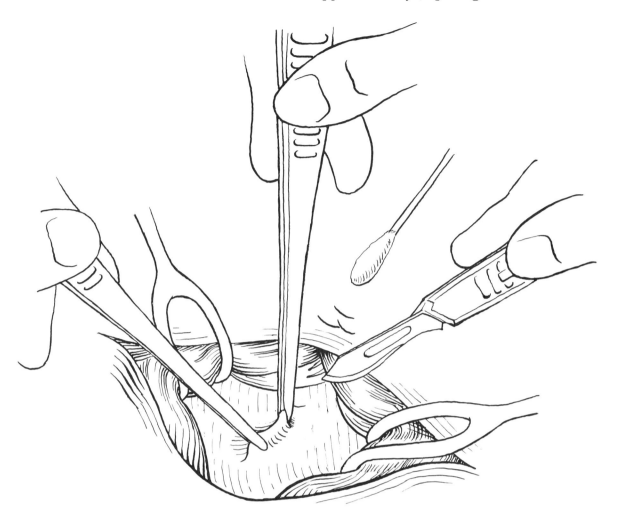

Fig. 13.9   Laparotomy pads are placed over all exposed
subcutaneous tissue. The peritoneum will often appear
inflamed, reflecting the underlying process. A small bite of the
peritoneum is picked up with forceps. DeBakey tissue forceps
are shown here. The assistant picks up a similar bite opposite
the surgeon. The surgeon releases and replaces his forceps
until he is satisfied that only the peritoneum is elevated.

Culture swabs (for aerobic and anaerobic culture) and
suction are held ready as a tiny nick is made in the peritoneum.
It is best to time this nick with expiration; the viscera can fall
away from the abdominal wall and air can enter the peritoneal
cavity.

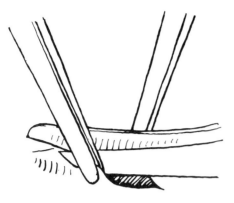

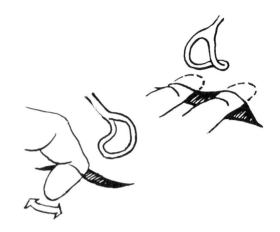

Fig. 13.10   The edges of the peritoneum are grasped and elevated. The blade of a Metzenbaum scissors is introduced, ideally under direct vision, and a clean cut is made. The peritoneum need not be opened to the full length of the skin incision since peritoneum stretches.

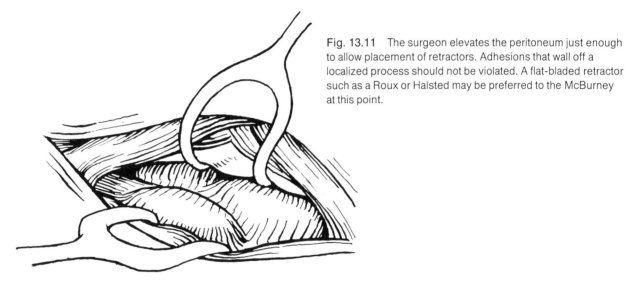

Fig. 13.11   The surgeon elevates the peritoneum just enough to allow placement of retractors. Adhesions that wall off a localized process should not be violated. A flat-bladed retractor such as a Roux or Halsted may be preferred to the McBurney at this point.

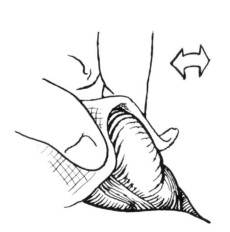

Fig. 13.12   The cecum is identified by its taeniae. The taenia is the strongest muscular part of the cecal wall. Hooking a finger under a taenia is frequently the easiest way to deliver the cecum into the operative field. Once the cecum is elevated, the left hand of the surgeon obtains a broad grasp with a moist pad. Gentle traction and a side-to-side rocking motion may deliver the appendix if it is not bound down. The three taeniae converge at the base of the appendix. Note that up to this point intraperitoneal manipulation has not been necessary.

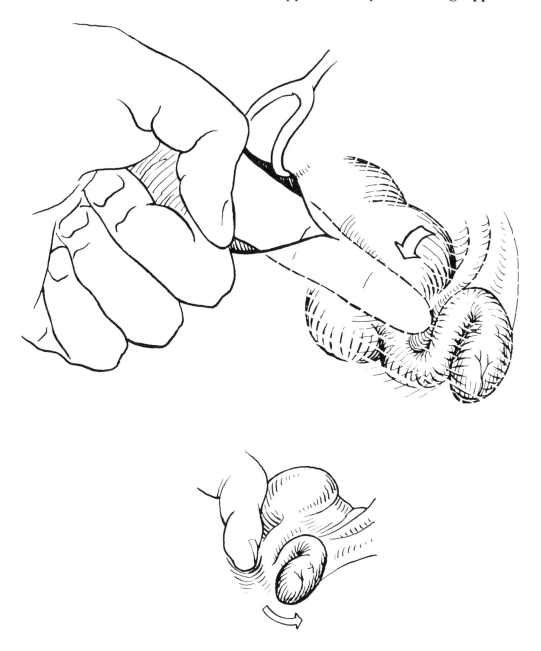

If the appendix is normal, one must think of the other common conditions that can mimic appendicitis: perforated peptic ulcer, terminal ileitis, Meckel's diverticulitis, gynecological pathology, cecal carcinoma (in the older patient), a perforated diverticulum, or diverticulitis and cholecystitis. Peritoneal fluid may be Gram stained and mesenteric lymph nodes can be examined. The appropriate steps, including laparotomy if indicated, must be taken until the diagnosis is made.

Fig. 13.13 If the appendix is not easily delivered, the surgeon explores carefully with his finger. This may be easier if the retractors are temporarily removed. The finger follows the anterolateral peritoneal surface and slowly sweeps away fibrinous adhesions from lateral to medial. Knowledge that the mesoappendix lies medially allows him to safely follow this approach. The appendix is gradually mobilized until the tip can be felt and delivered. Sometimes this maneuver requires a great deal of patience and skill.

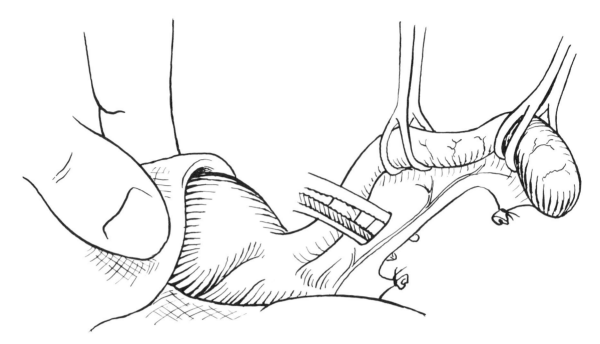

Fig. 13.14 The appendix is gently elevated to stretch its mesentery. Babcock clamps surround the appendix and clamp on the mesentery in this illustration. An alternative is to clamp the free edge of the mesentery below the tip of the appendix. The appendix should be touched and manipulated as little as possible to avoid spreading contamination.

Holding the cecum rather than dropping it back at this point provides control of the appendiceal stump and artery. The wound edges – including all layers of the abdominal wall – are protected by moist laparotomy pads.

Palpation of the mesoappendix reveals the location of the main appendiceal artery. As in all extirpative surgery, the blood supply is taken first. Transillumination by the overhead lights is the most precise and elegant way of localizing vessels but may be unsuccessful because of inflammatory thickening of the mesoappendix. If successful, however, it obviates touching the mesoappendix.

A hole is created with clamp tips near the base of the mesoappendix, isolating a narrow band of tissue with one or two vessels. The clamp is spread gently parallel to the vessels to provide room for tying without tearing adjacent vessels or appendix. The segment is clamped, divided, and ligated as described in Chapter 5. The mesentery is serially divided to the base of the appendix. It is often wise to doubly ligate or suture ligate the appendiceal artery while it is in view. The elastic vessel tends to retract deep into the mesentery if it escapes.

Time should be taken to tie the appendiceal side of the clamped mesentery rather than leaving the clamps attached to cause unnecessary tension on the appendix.

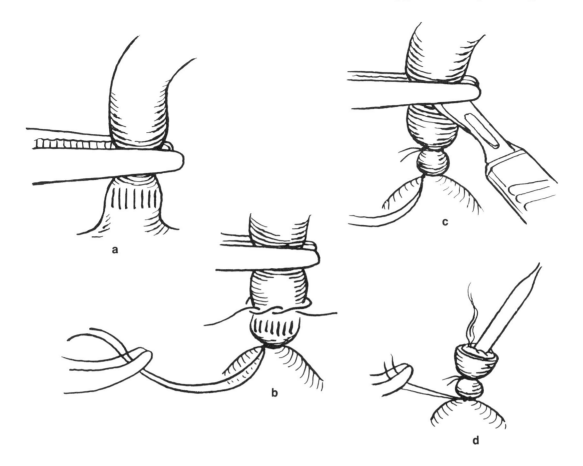

Fig. 13.15 The appendiceal base is crushed with a straight or right-angle clamp just above its junction with cecum **a**). The clamp is released and the appendix distal to this point is gently milked to displace contaminated contents and fecolith if present. The appendix is doubly ligated with 2–0 chromic suture at the upper and lower margins of the crush marks **b**) while being held by a clamp a few millimeters distal to the second tie. The appendix is sharply divided on the proximal side of the clamp while the long ends of the first tie are held for control **c**). The contaminated knife and the appendix are passed off the field. The exposed lumen may then be cauterized with the Bovie or with phenol and alcohol. **d**) It may also be left untouched.

The stump may also be handled by inversion and purse-string suture or Z-stitch. It is preferable not to tie the stump first if this is done so that an isolated segment of lumen cannot progress to abscess or mucocele. A tied, inverted stump may persist as a mass and be hard to differentiate from a cecal tumor at a later time.

A very necrotic stump may require inversion or even temporary tube cecostomy for safe management. If tube cecostomy is done, the cecal wall must be secured to the peritoneum at the site of the cecostomy.

The stump and cecum should be thoroughly lavaged with saline (some use antibiotic solution). Contaminated instruments and suction should not be used again.

In a simple appendectomy, the benefit of running the terminal ileum for other pathology must be weighed against the possibility of spreading of contamination.

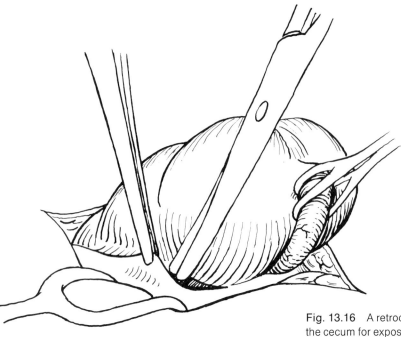

Fig. 13.16   A retrocecal appendix may require mobilization of the cecum for exposure. The lateral attachment of the cecum along the avascular "white line" is sharply divided. The cecum is elevated, and the appendix is carefully delivered and excised.

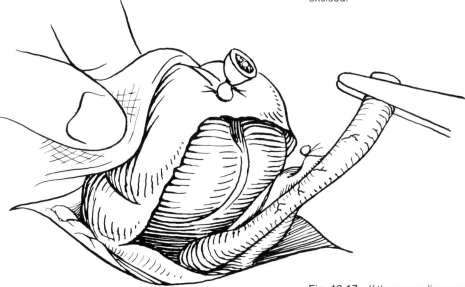

Fig. 13.17   If the appendix cannot be safety delivered without risk of rupture, retrograde (in relation to the cecum) excision may be carried out. The origin of the mesentery should be kept in mind as the vessels are divided. It is vitally important to work under direct vision. A blindly exploring finger in this location can easily mistake the ureter for the appendix.

If the tip is still difficult to reach, do not hestitate to extend the incision for adequate exposure. The young surgeon sometimes loses perspective in such a struggle. The attending surgeon's first suggestion on entering the room is invariably to lengthen the incision.

Unless there is a well-developed abscess cavity from a perforated appendix, there is no indication for a drain. A drain in the free peritoneal cavity is walled off in 8–12 hours.

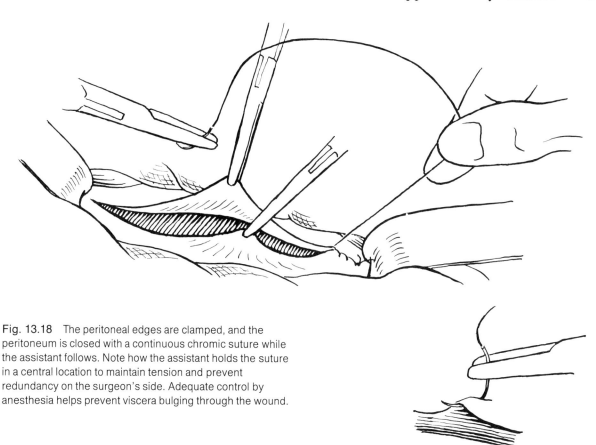

Fig. 13.18 The peritoneal edges are clamped, and the peritoneum is closed with a continuous chromic suture while the assistant follows. Note how the assistant holds the suture in a central location to maintain tension and prevent redundancy on the surgeon's side. Adequate control by anesthesia helps prevent viscera bulging through the wound.

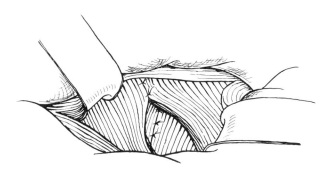

Fig. 13.19 The muscles are closed in layers. Small bites of the strong outer fascial layer of the transversus and internal oblique muscles give effective closure. The overlapping layers provide added strength to the closure. Absorbable suture can be used for all layers.

Irrigation after closure of each layer is beneficial. This serves to mechanically debride loose particles and dilutes bacteria to the point of extinction. Sponging the fluid with a clean laparotomy pad may pick up more debris than using the suction.

Subcutaneous tissue is lavaged; Scarpa's fascia and skin may be closed in a minimally contaminated case.

In the face of gross soilage, leave the wound open and close it secondarily in a few days.

Once these details become automatic you will find that an uncomplicated appendectomy can easily be done in half an hour without rushing. Great satisfaction is derived from doing even the most simple case well.

Chapter 14

Inguinal Hernia

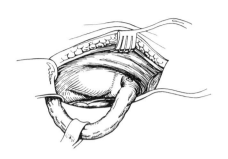

Preparation of the patient for herniorrhaphy requires thorough preoperative evaluation for conditions that increase intra-abdominal pressure. Such conditions as obstructive genitourinary, colonic, or pulmonary disease predispose a patient to early failure of the repair. The patient must be thoroughly informed about what to expect if local anesthesia is elected. He must also know what physical restrictions he will observe in the postoperative period.

The second major requirement for a smooth surgical procedure is a knowledgeable surgeon. Few areas of human anatomy are as misunderstood as the inguinal region. A solid understanding of three-dimensional relationships is essential to effect a lasting repair. The first part of this chapter is an attempt to clarify inguinal anatomy.

Good judgment superimposed on thorough anatomical knowledge dictates the surgeon's response to the kind of hernia and the strength of the tissues. A logical progression (e.g., checking for indirect, di-

rect, and femoral hernias, in order) prevents omission of important steps.

The third component of a rigorous approach to a surgical procedure involves the principles of technique outlined earlier. Be aware of these principles throughout the following presentation. Attention to details of technique can avoid major problems later. An insecure knot on the superficial epigastric artery can lead to a postoperative hematoma. The hematoma, which is an excellent culture medium, can become infected and form an abscess. The infection leads to fascial necrosis and the repair breaks down. The patient suffers a prolonged recovery period and requires a second operation. It would have been much easier if the surgeon took the care to tie a good knot.

Keep in mind that these principles are interdependent. One without the others is useless. Adopt a unified approach to your surgery.

Anatomy

Both the clinical importance and anatomical complexity of the inguinal region are disproportionate to its size. In this very small area one finds a conjunction of structures belonging to the abdominal wall, pelvis, and lower extremity. The inguinal ligament is a key structure that will serve as a reference point in describing inguinal anatomy. This ligament consists of the most caudal aponeurotic fibers of the external oblique muscle that form a bridge between the anterior superior spine of the ilium and the pubic tubercle (Fig. 14.1). The bulk of the space beneath its span is filled laterally by the iliopsoas muscle mass. Medially, fibers of the inguinal ligament recurve toward the pectineal ligament (the thickened periosteum over the pectineal line of the pubis, also called Cooper's ligament to form the lacunar ligament. Between the edge of the lacunar ligament and the muscle mass is a space through which the iliac artery, iliac vein, and femoral nerve pass. The vessels, however, are not in direct contact with the bordering structures, and this fact is critical to the understanding of the pathogenesis of femoral hernia.

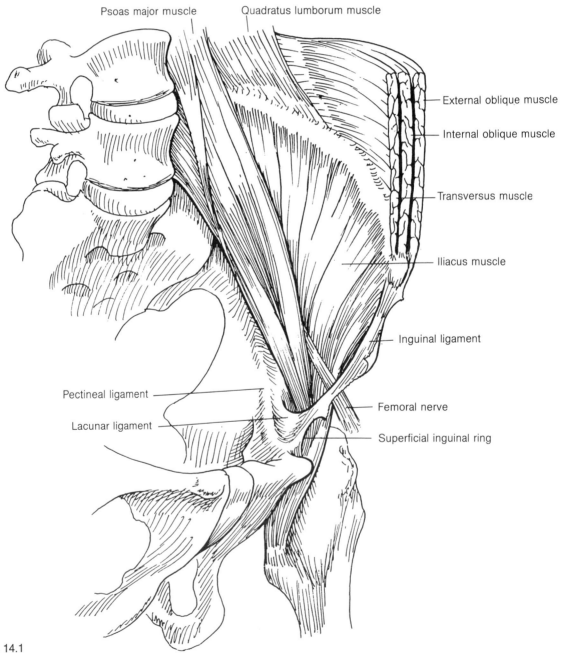

Psoas major muscle

Quadratus lumborum muscle

External oblique muscle

Internal oblique muscle

Transversus muscle

Iliacus muscle

Inguinal ligament

Pectineal ligament

Femoral nerve

Lacunar ligament

Superficial inguinal ring

Fig. 14.1

The vessels passing beneath the inguinal ligament are enclosed by a continuation of the transversalis fascia, which lines the entire abdominal cavity (Fig. 14.2). This fascial evagination forms a femoral sheath that continues a short distance into the thigh. Between the femoral vein and the portion of the sheath covering the edge of the lacunar ligament, a potential space exists through which abdominal contents can protrude. Because of the narrowness of the opening and the unyielding nature of the surrounding structures, such a hernia has a tendency to incarcerate and strangulate its contents. The transversalis fascia is closely applied to the underside of the transversus abdominis muscle and its continuation caudal to that muscle is the main constituent of the posterior wall of the inguinal canal.

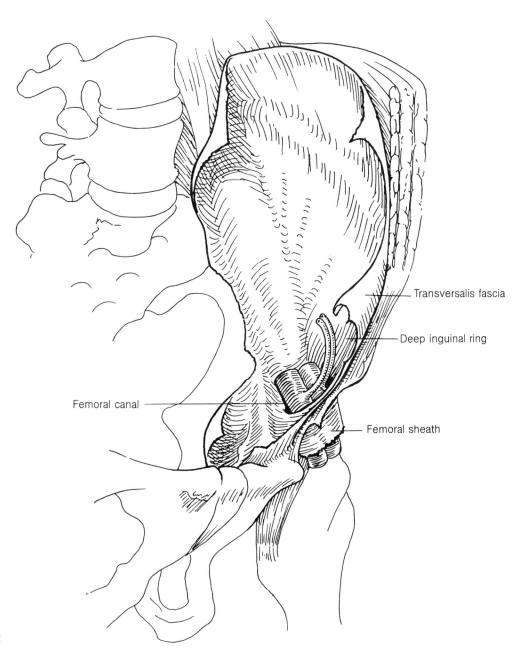

Transversalis fascia

Deep inguinal ring

Femoral canal

Femoral sheath

Fig. 14.2

The muscular fibers of the internal oblique and transversus muscles end cephalad to the inguinal ligament (Fig. 14.3). The transversalis fascia is continuous below the arch formed by the edge of these muscles and is loosely bound to the part of the inguinal ligament forming the floor of the inguinal canal. The fascia then continues posteriorly to pass over the pectineal ligament into the pelvis. The caudad edge of the transversus muscle is aponeurotic and intimately adherent to transversalis fascia. This transversus aponeurosis arch is the key structure used for all types of inguinal hernia repair. The medial portions of internal oblique and transversus muscles fuse into a true "conjoined tendon" in a relatively small proportion of people prior to blending into the anterior rectus sheath. Note that the external oblique aponeurosis joins the rectus sheath more medially than the other two muscles.

The spermatic cord penetrates the transversalis fascia lateral to the inferior epigastric vessels, forming the deep inguinal ring and taking a covering of transversalis fascia called the internal spermatic fascia. When abdominal contents and peritoneum protrude within this layer, it is called an indirect inguinal hernia. A protrusion through the transversalis fascia covering the space medial to these vessels (Hesselbach's triangle) is a direct inguinal hernia. The cord receives a covering of cremasteric muscle and fascia from the internal oblique muscle and then traverses the inguinal canal, which is bounded by the transversalis fascia posteriorly, the external oblique aponeurosis anteriorly, and the inguinal ligament inferiorly. The cord exits the inguinal canal at the pubic tubercle where the fibers of the external oblique aponeurosis split to form the superficial inguinal ring. A final fascial contribution to the cord from the investing fascia on the external oblique aponeurosis forms the thin external spermatic fascia.

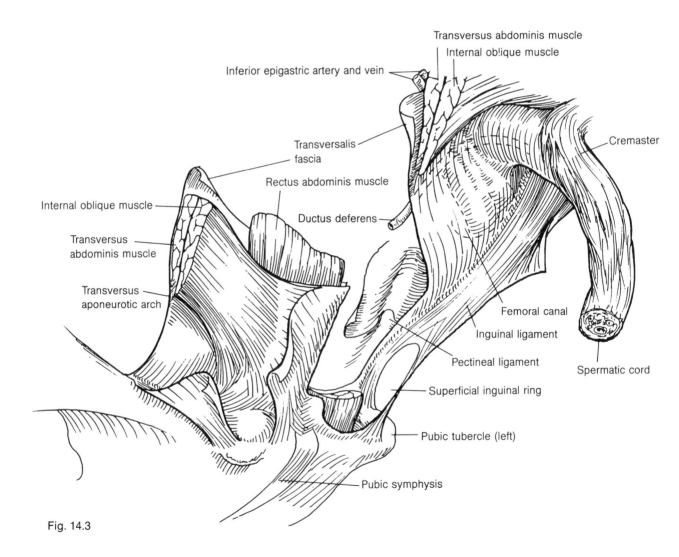

Fig. 14.3

The structures wrapped within the layers of the spermatic cord are the ductus deferens, the internal spermatic vessels, and the genitofemoral nerve (Fig. 14.4). The ductus deferens rises from the pelvis and crosses the iliac vessels posterior to the inferior epigastric artery and vein to reach the deep ring. The spermatic vessels descend from their upper abdominal origins (aorta, vena cava, and left renal vein) and are joined by the genitofemoral nerve and, finally, the ductus deferens at the deep ring. The view from the cephalad direction demonstrates the validity of the alternate preperitoneal approach to repair of inguinal and femoral hernias.

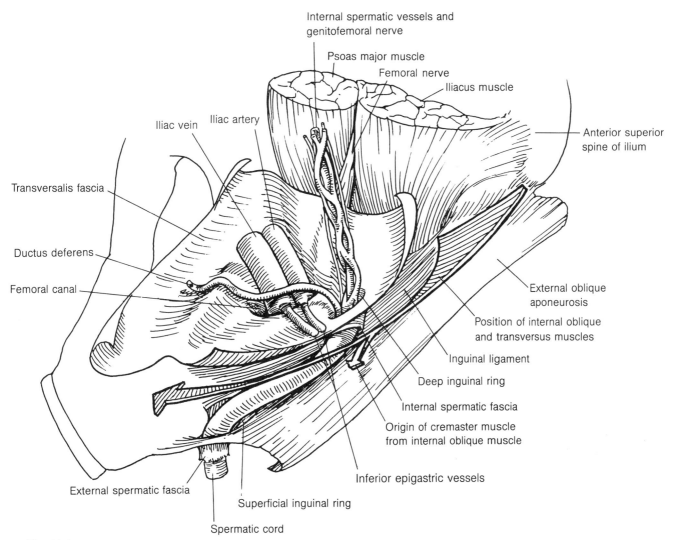

Fig. 14.4

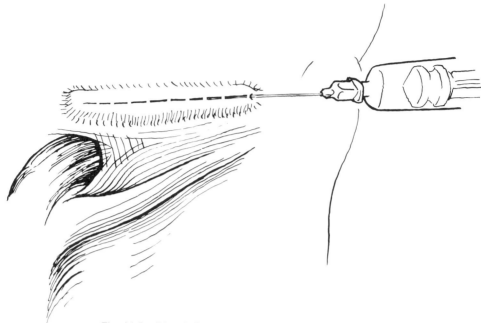

Fig. 14.5   Direct infiltration and field block are two methods of administering local anesthesia. The former is depicted here. Pre-op sedation should be timed to be fully effective when the skin incision is made. There is a variety of suitable drug combinations; choice should be dictated by the patient's age and condition.

Local Anesthesia

At the Shouldice Hospital in Toronto, a total of up to 150 ml of 2% procaine without epinephrine is routinely used. Adequate anesthesia can be accomplished with considerably less – for example, 50 ml of 1% lidocaine without epinephrine – decreasing the threat for systemic toxicity posed by the higher dose.

An intradermal injection along the line of incision raises a wheal and immediately anesthetizes skin. A 22-g spinal needle is suitable for infiltration. Injection should be done slowly because it is the sudden stretch of the tissues that is sensed as pain. Injection is made while both advancing and withdrawing the needle. It is not necessary to aspirate because the time the needle is in any blood vessel is insignificant.

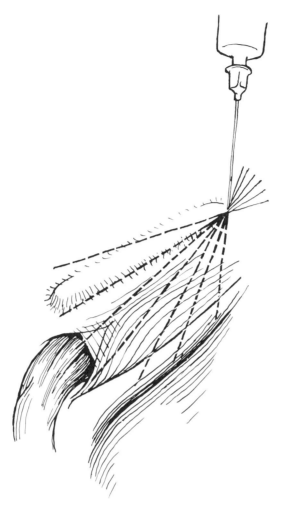

Fig. 14.6   The needle is withdrawn and reinserted
subcutaneously in a fanlike pattern. It must be withdrawn
almost to the skin in order to redirect it. Bending a partially
withdrawn shaft leaves the needle in the same tract. Care is
taken to inject cephalad and at the ends of the proposed
incision.

The superficial layers usually require about 30 ml
of anesthetic. An additional amount is injected beneath the intact external oblique aponeurosis to
block the ilioinguinal nerve. A supplemental injection is made at the deep ring prior to pulling on the
peritoneum. Injection around the pubic tubercle before mobilizing the cord is helpful.

Fig. 14.7   The skin incision may be parallel with and cephalad to the inguinal ligament, or more transverse to parallel skin lines. The lower edge of the inguinal ligament lies a few centimeters cephalad to the inguinal crease. Skin traction, applied with the flattened hands of surgeon and assistant, is increased as the tissues are incised and begin to yield. Significant skin bleeders are secured. Retractors (rakes shown here) are positioned and gently pulled apart and upward.

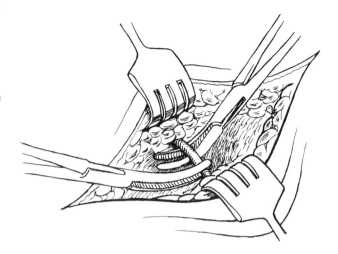

By proceeding carefully with the second knife, the surgeon can identify and expose one or two major subcutaneous vessels before they are cut. The superficial epigastric vessels are the ones usually encountered in the center of the incision. They are isolated, clamped, divided, and ligated. Frequently a second significant vessel, a branch of the superficial circumflex iliac, is found laterally.

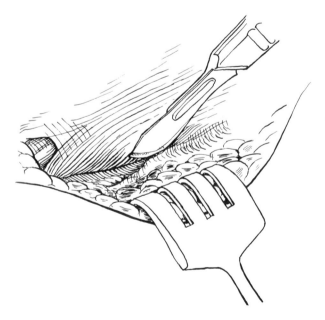

Fig. 14.8   Scarpa's fascia is incised the full length of the incision, exposing the external oblique aponeurosis. Unnecessary subcutaneous undermining creates a large dead space. The fine network of vessels on the surface of the external oblique aponeurosis is disturbed as little as possible. This is the blood supply of the fascia. The superficial ring with its intercrural fiber bridge is now visualized. The reflected edge of the inguinal ligament is sharply exposed by dividing the investing fascia while the assistant increases traction on the lower retractor.

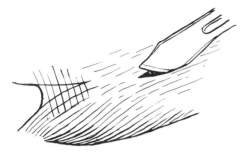

Fig. 14.9   A nick is made in external oblique aponeurosis. (Extra protection is afforded to the ilioinguinal nerve if local anesthesia is injected beneath the external oblique layer prior to opening.)

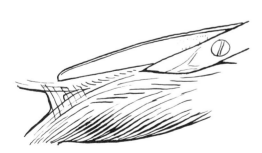

Fig. 14.10   A Metzenbaum scissors is passed toward the superficial ring immediately beneath the aponeurosis, with the points held closed and up.

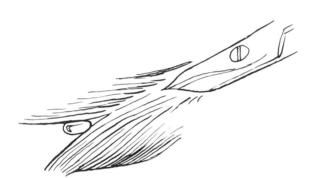

Fig. 14.11   The scissors is withdrawn and turned 90°, and one blade is inserted the full length of the intended cut. A single smooth cut is made. Shearing by pushing a partially opened scissors is more traumatic than cutting.

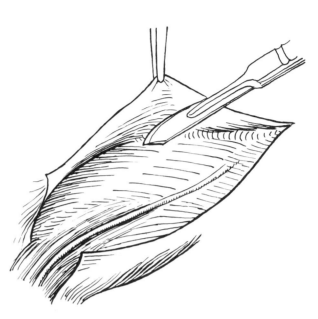

Fig. 14.12   The superior (medial) flap of the external oblique aponeurosis is elevated from the internal oblique, preferably by sharp dissection.

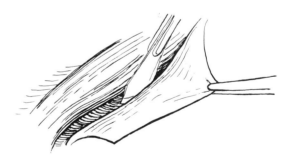

Fig. 14.13   The lateral flap is developed, exposing the reflected or shelving edge of the inguinal ligament. A broad-bladed retractor such as a Roux may be placed medially and laterally beneath the external oblique layer. Wound edges should be protected with pads to prevent desiccation and contamination.

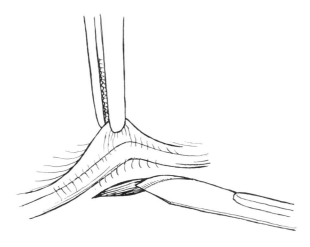

Fig. 14.14   The ilioinguinal nerve, originating predominantly from L1, innervates abdominal muscles along its course and provides sensory innervation to the skin of the pubis and upper scrotum. It is consistently found on the anterior surface of the cremaster layer, overlying the spermatic cord. Injury to this nerve can cause considerable postoperative discomfort. Occasionally a hypogastric branch of the iliohypogastric nerve will also be found within the inguinal canal.

The ilioinguinal nerve lies within a loose fascial plane. The adjacent fascia is grasped so that the nerve can be elevated and the fascia incised. The nerve should never be grasped directly.

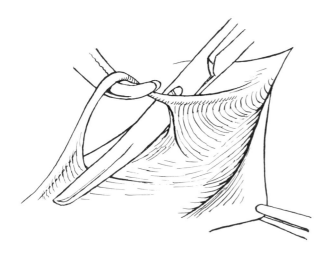

Fig. 14.15   An opening is made in the fascia, and the nerve is gently elevated without stretching. The tented fascia can then be cut close to the nerve in both directions. A significant bleeding point may be encountered, usually on the proximal side. This should be precisely clamped with a fine mosquito (Halsted) clamp and carefully ligated as far from the nerve as possible. Never cauterize near a nerve because the transmitted heat or current may cause injury.

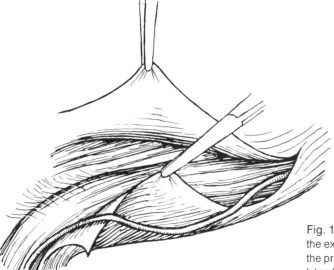

Fig. 14.16   The mobilized nerve is displaced outside one of the external oblique flaps for protection during the remainder of the procedure. A self-retaining retractor may then be placed laterally.

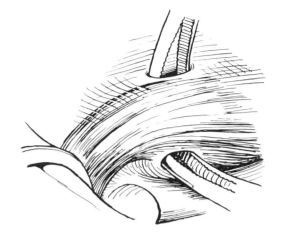

Fig. 14.17   At the pubic tubercle there is a plane between the cord and internal oblique. The cord is isolated by careful dissection with blunt clamps. Blunt dissection by the surgeon's fingers can be quite traumatic. A Penrose drain is passed beneath the cord for traction.

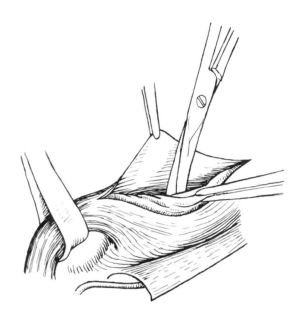

Fig. 14.18   The cremaster muscle is opened anteriorly in the line of its fibers. This muscle does not completely encircle the cord. It is absent on the posterior surface. Flaps are dissected medially and laterally. Traction and countertraction are essential to good dissection.

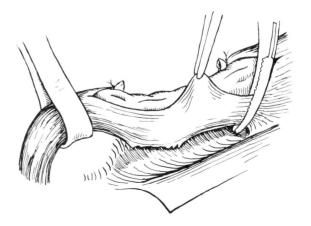

Fig. 14.19   The centers of the flaps are separated from the inguinal floor and the segments of cremaster, excised between clamps. This maneuver exposes the floor of the inguinal canal and allows a more accurate repair. Some surgeons may choose not to excise the cremaster in the face of a simple indirect hernia. There is no significant morbidity associated with taking the cremaster.

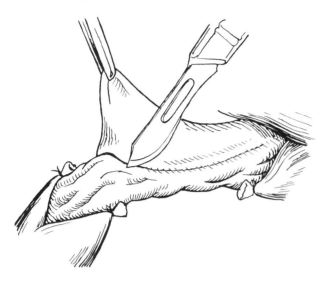

Fig. 14.20   The cord is now inspected for an indirect hernia sac, which should be found anteromedially. If a sac is found, it is gently elevated to define its borders. The avascular plane between sac and cord should be sharply incised until the sac is free down to the deep ring. Opening the fundus of the sac and inserting a finger may facilitate the dissection. The assistant applies countertraction to the adjacent cord with atraumatic forceps.

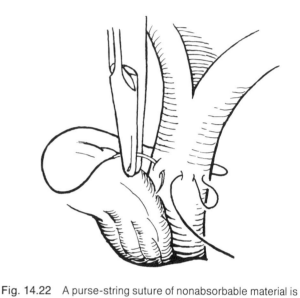

Fig. 14.22   A purse-string suture of nonabsorbable material is placed under direct vision as the sac is gently pulled. The suture is tied and a second tie may be placed. The end of the suture is left long for control of the stump.

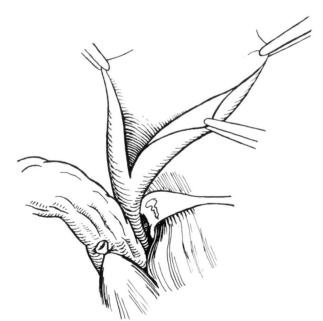

Fig. 14.21   The sac is opened on its medial side to avoid injuring viscera in case there is a sliding hernia. A finger is now inserted into the peritoneal cavity to check the direct space and femoral canal. Note that the arching fibers of the internal oblique and transversus muscles at the superior rim of the deep ring are retracted for exposure.

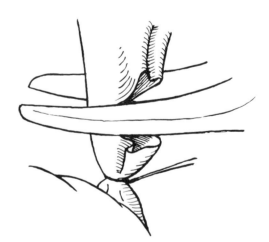

Fig. 14.23   The excess sac is excised with a heavy scissors; then the suture is cut. The stump should retract out of sight.

Techniques of Repair

The two types of repair shown in the following illustrations are proven and anatomically sound. One is the transversalis/iliopubic tract repair represented by the Shouldice technique. The other is the Cooper's ligament repair represented by the McVay technique. Both depend on the transversus aponeurosis/transversalis fascial layer for reconstructing the floor. Preparation of this layer (shown in Figs. 14.24 through 14.33) is common to both types of repair.

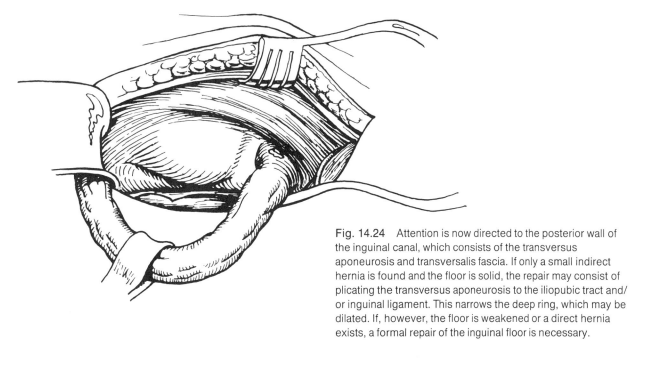

Fig. 14.24　Attention is now directed to the posterior wall of the inguinal canal, which consists of the transversus aponeurosis and transversalis fascia. If only a small indirect hernia is found and the floor is solid, the repair may consist of plicating the transversus aponeurosis to the iliopubic tract and/or inguinal ligament. This narrows the deep ring, which may be dilated. If, however, the floor is weakened or a direct hernia exists, a formal repair of the inguinal floor is necessary.

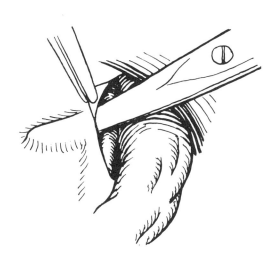

Fig. 14.25　The transversalis layer is carefully opened at the medial edge of the deep ring. A scissors is insinated between the transversalis fascia and inferior epigastric vessels. The transversalis layer is opened down to the pubic tubercle.

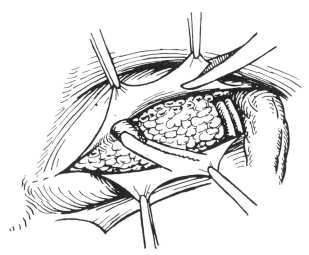

Fig. 14.26　The flaps are elevated, and preperitoneal fat is swept off the undersurface of transversalis. The caudad flap is commonly referred to as the lateral flap and the cephalad flap as the medial flap because of their oblique relationship. The pubic branch of the inferior epigastric vessels lies under the lateral flap; care must be taken not to avulse these vessels in clearing the flap. The weakened transversalis fascia is excised from both flaps.

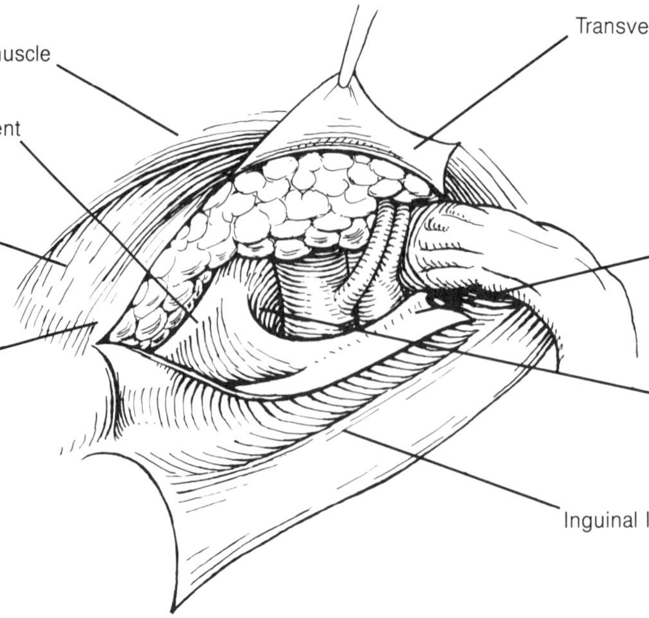

Internal oblique muscle

Transversalis fascia

Pectineal (Cooper's) ligament

Transversus muscle

Iliopubic tract

Transversus aponeurosis

Femoral canal

Inguinal ligament

Fig. 14.27   A more cephalad view with the transversalis layer opened shows the relationship of the internal oblique, transversus muscle, transversus aponeurosis, and transversalis fascia (above) to the inguinal ligament, iliopubic tract, Cooper's ligament, and femoral canal (below). Note that the lateral flap of the transversalis is still adherent to the lower edge of inguinal ligament. Cooper's ligament can be seen from the cephalad view but not from an anterior view.

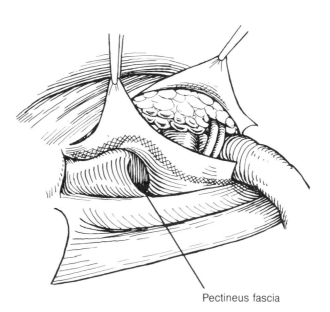

Pectineus fascia

Fig. 14.28   The connection between the transversalis fascia (specifically iliopubic tract) and inguinal ligament has been broken, and the transversalis has been elevated off the lacunar ligament, revealing the transversalis attachment to Cooper's ligament. This view also demonstrates why the rim of the femoral sheath, and not the edge of the lacunar ligament, forms the medial margin of the femoral canal. The iliopubic tract is crosshatched. Remember that there is variability in the strength of the iliopubic tract just as there is in the transversus aponeurosis.

The pectineus fascia can be seen beneath the rim of the lacunar ligament.

Fig. 14.29   The transversus abdominis arch and the lateral flap of the transversalis have now been prepared for either type of repair previously alluded to on page 225. The vertical line represents the plane of the sagittal section shown in Fig. 14.30.

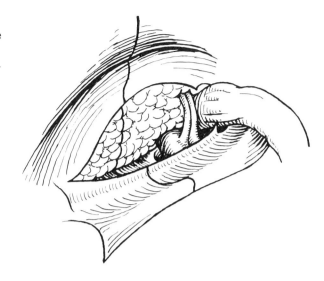

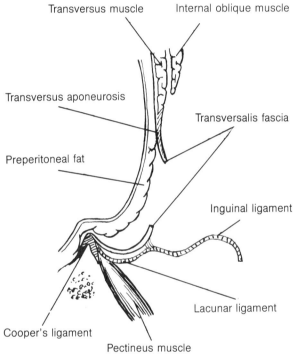

Transversus muscle   Internal oblique muscle

Transversus aponeurosis

Transversalis fascia

Preperitoneal fat

Inguinal ligament

Cooper's ligament

Lacunar ligament

Pectineus muscle

Fig. 14.30   The relationship between layers can now be seen.

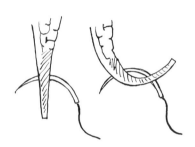

Fig. 14.31   The shaded area represents the transversus aponeurosis fusing with the transversalis fascia. This layer may be taken with a simple suture or with a suture through the reflected undersurface. The latter approach allows the free edge to be used for a second layer.

The two types of repair shown in the following illustrations are proven and anatomically sound. One is the transversalis/iliopubic tract repair represented by the Shouldice technique. the other is the Cooper's ligament repair represented by the McVay technique. Both depend on the transversus aponeurosis/transversalis fascial layer for reconstructing the floor. Preparation of this layer (shown in Figs. 12.24 through 12.32) is common to both types of repair.

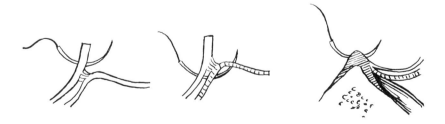

Fig. 14.32   The iliopubic tract may be taken alone or with the shelving edge of the inguinal ligament for the lateral bite. In the alternate repair of the inguinal floor, the lateral bite is taken through Cooper's ligament.

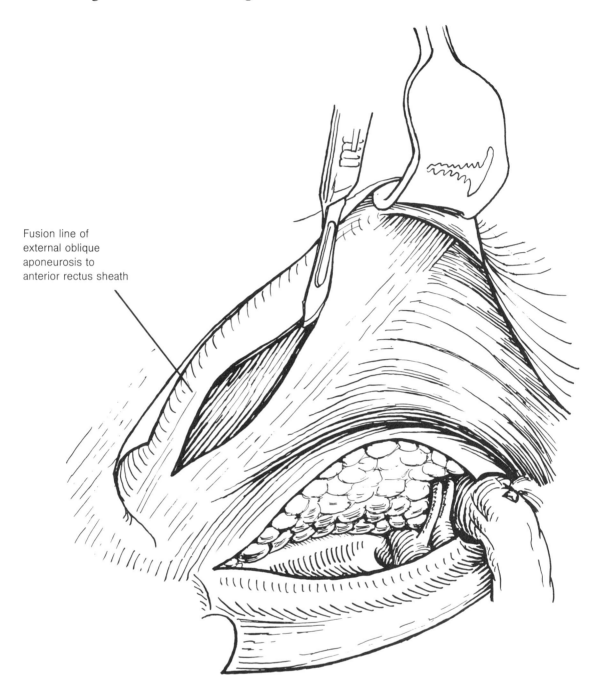

Fusion line of
external oblique
aponeurosis to
anterior rectus sheath

Fig. 14.33 Controversy exists regarding the necessity of a "relaxing" incision in the anterior rectus sheath. This is made lateral to the fusion of the external oblique aponeurosis. Proponents feel that it facilitates bringing the transversus abdominis arch down to the iliopubic tract (Condon) or Cooper's ligament (McVay) without tension. Advocates of the Shouldice repair (which sutures the transversus abdominis arch to the iliopubic tract and inguinal ligament) rarely if ever use a relaxing incision. Since local anesthesia is generally used with this repair, an accurate appreciation of true tension can be gained at the operating table. This procedure has a lower recurrence rate than does the Cooper's ligament repair.

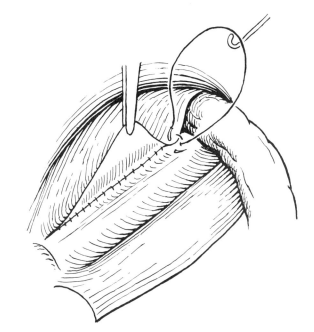

Fig. 14.34 This figure represents the use of the iliopubic tract and inguinal ligament to anchor the repair.

The Shouldice repair uses continuous No. 34 monofilament stainless steel wire. A first row starts at the pubic tubercule, and the reflected edge of the medial flap is sutured down to the lateral flap of the transversalis (iliopubic tract). At the deep ring the suture is reversed, and the free edge of the medial flap is sutured to the inguinal ligament. The ends are tied at the pubic tubercle. Another double row is placed between the transversus abdominis arch and inguinal ligament to complete the repair.

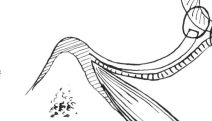

Fig. 14.35 This cross section shows the two components of the first double layer of the Shouldice repair.

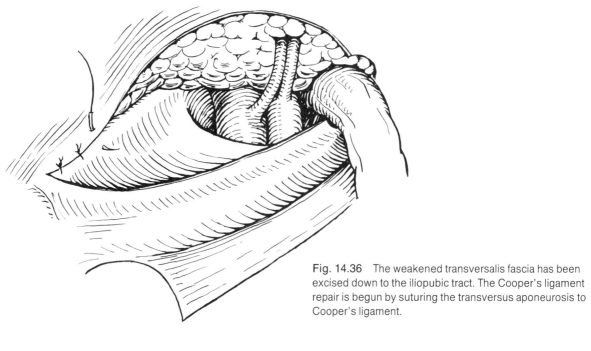

Fig. 14.36   The weakened transversalis fascia has been excised down to the iliopubic tract. The Cooper's ligament repair is begun by suturing the transversus aponeurosis to Cooper's ligament.

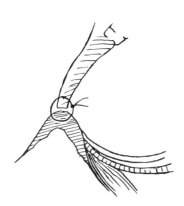

Fig. 14.37   This is a cross section of the medial part of the Cooper's ligament repair.

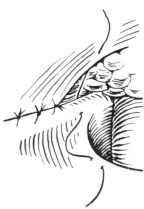

Fig. 14.38   At the femoral vessels a "transition stitch" sutures the transversus aponeurosis to Cooper's ligament, the pectineus fascia, and the medial margin of the anterior femoral sheath. This stitch bridges the gap, which can be up to 2 cm wide, between Cooper's ligament and the inguinal ligament.

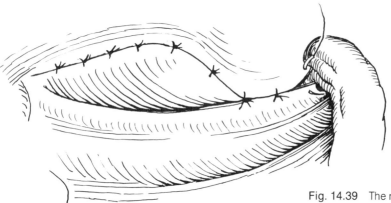

Fig. 14.39   The repair is completed by suturing the remaining transversus aponeurosis to the anterior femoral sheath.

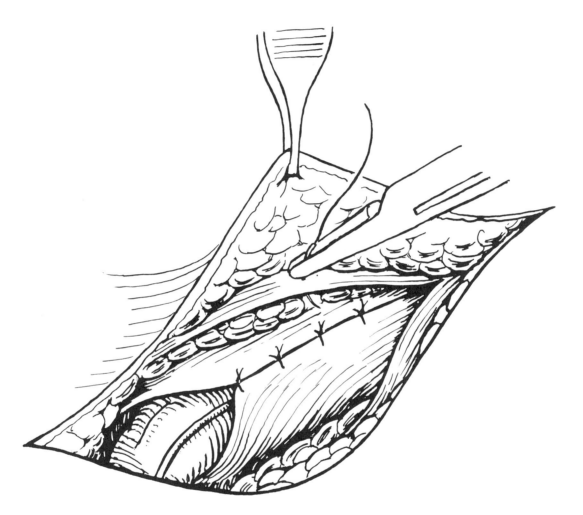

Fig. 14.40   The wound is thoroughly lavaged with saline, the ilioinguinal nerve and cord are replaced in their anatomical positions, and the external oblique is loosely closed. Scarpa's fascia is tensed by gently lifting straight up on skin. The fascia is then easily approximated. The skin can be closed with sutures or with clips.

Chapter 15

Cholecystectomy

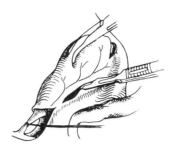

Cholecystectomy is frequently the first major abdominal procedure performed by the junior surgical resident. The resident might assume that it is first because he can do little harm, and might consequently approach the case without the proper respect for the danger involved. In fact, injury to the common duct often results in suffering and death for the patient.

Patients with gallbladder disease often are obese and have a deep, inaccessible common duct. In addition to observing all the other elements of good surgery, the surgeon must pay particular attention to exposure and identification of structures in this procedure.

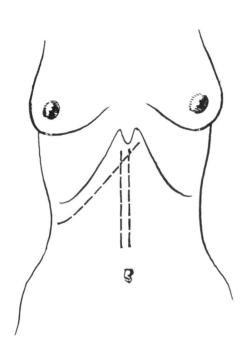

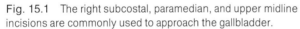

Fig. 15.1   The right subcostal, paramedian, and upper midline incisions are commonly used to approach the gallbladder.

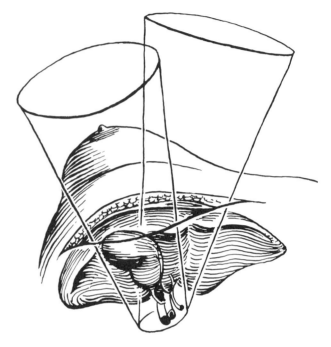

Fig. 15.2   Optimal lighting for a cholecystectomy is obtained by directing the lights cephalad and medially. One light directly overhead (the opposite light in a two-track system) and one directed over the surgeon's right shoulder best accomplish this.

The major force of the abdominal muscles is transverse. Many surgeons feel that a transverse incision heals better for this reason and that the patient has less discomfort with the subcostal incision, which also gives excellent exposure. The advocates of vertical incisions argue correctly that the common duct is a midline structure. Also, these incisions can be extended if lower abdominal pathology is encountered. In addition, intercostal nerves are not cut and the vertical incisions are made more quickly than the subcostal one.

Most operating room lights can be adjusted in intensity and focus. The more narrowly the beam is focused, the greater is the spot illumination. An adhesive plastic drape can be used to immobilize residual skin bacteria; it also eliminates the need for towel clips, which might interfere with x-ray films.

The patient should be on a table suitable for x-ray studies. The x-ray technician should have positioned the first cassette and taken a scout film prior to the start of the procedure.

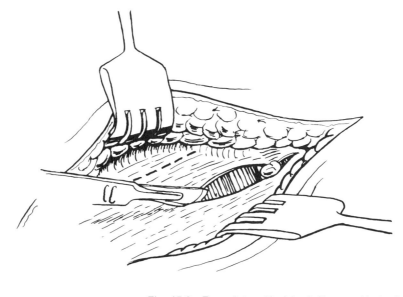

Fig. 15.3   The subcostal incision is illustrated in the following drawings. The generous skin incision is started across the midline almost at the opposite costal margin. It is rapidly carried down to fascia along its entire length. Hemostasis is then accomplished as previously described. The incision must be kept parallel to and at least 3 cm from the costal margin (*dotted line*) to allow adequate tissue for closure. An incisional hernia at the costal margin is difficult to repair.

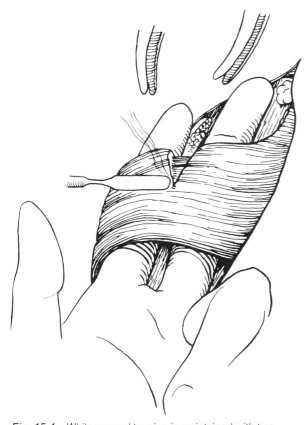

When the anterior rectus sheath is incised, a button of preperitoneal fat will appear to identify the midline. A T-shaped extension at the lateral edge of the rectus sheath facilitates insertion of the fingers to elevate the rectus muscle.

Electrocoagulation causes considerable muscular contraction and should be kept at the lowest effective current. Periodic release of tension identifies vessels in the cut edges, which can then be individually clamped and ligated. Gross clamping across the body of the muscle should be avoided.

The blood supply of the rectus muscle originates in the superior and inferior epigastric vessels.

Fig. 15.4   While upward tension is maintained with two fingers of the surgeon's left hand, the rectus muscle is gradually divided by electrocoagulation (blended current) or knife. The blend mode adds a component of intermittent coagulating current to the continuous cutting current to achieve both purposes.

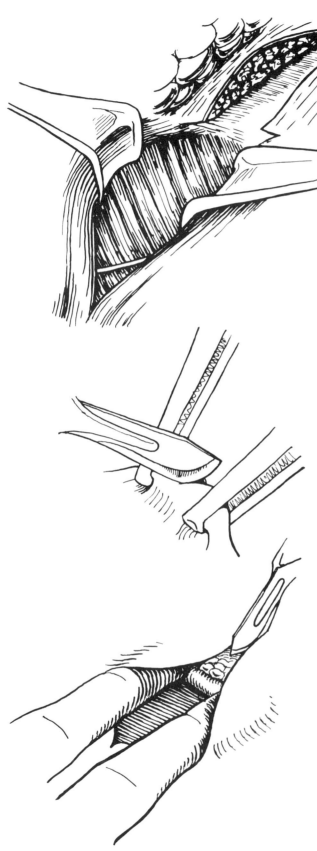

Fig. 15.5   The rectus muscle is innervated by intercostal nerves 7–12. The incision is extended far enough laterally to give good exposure while preserving as many intercostal nerves as possible. The nerves lie between the internal oblique and transversus muscles and are usually accompanied by small blood vessels. Damage to these vessels usually ends in clamping and dividing the nerve.

The flank muscles are divided along the lines of their fibers. For each layer, the superficial fascia of the muscle is incised rather than torn.

Fig. 15.6   A fold of posterior rectus sheath and peritoneum is elevated and carefully incised. When a clear opening is established, it is enlarged to allow introduction of two fingers.

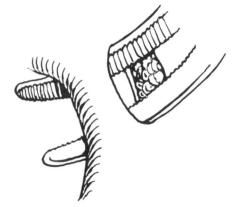

Fig. 15.7   Peritoneum and posterior rectus sheath are incised medially over the round ligament and laterally to the end of the incision.

Fig. 15.8   It is often possible to gain good exposure without dividing the round ligament. This depends on the habitus and anatomy of the patient. If the ligament is divided, it should be securely tied with heavy (2–0) suture material. The cut hepatic end can be clamped and used for traction to gain better exposure.

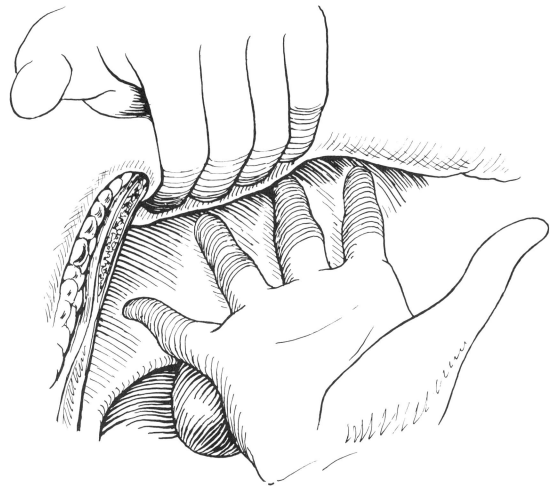

Fig. 15.9 When the incision is complete, the edge of the abdominal wall is protected with moist pads. The pads are placed with one hand while the opposite hand separates the viscera from the abdominal wall.

The right hand can be placed above the liver to let air enter between liver and diaphragm. This allows a high-riding liver to descend into the operative field. The maneuver is not always necessary or desirable (e.g., in the presence of gross infection).

In the course of systematic exploration, the pylorus and duodenal bulb are examined for scarring. The esophageal hiatus is probed and should feel snug to the fingertip. The pancreas is checked for induration and other signs of inflammation. Evaluation of the lower abdomen includes a check for diverticular disease. Exploration is not done in the presence of an abscess.

There are several long-armed self-retaining retractors available. If these are placed carefully, exposure can be improved without traumatizing tissue.

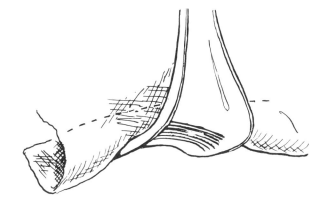

Fig. 15.10 Only enough pad to protect the wound is placed over the edge. Excess pad will fall down and impair exposure when the retractors are placed.

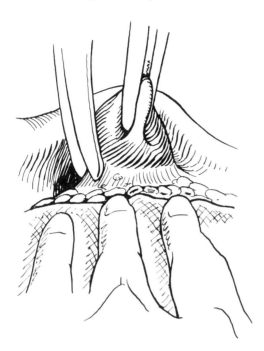

Fig. 15.11   The ability of the body to wall off an inflammatory process is an important defense mechanism. After repeated bouts of cholecystitis, the gallbladder is often found encased in omentum and adherent to the duodenum and colon. Careful sharp dissection should be kept close to the wall of the gallbladder to avoid injuring adjacent structures such as colon or duodenum. It may go slowly at first. Traction and countertraction must be maintained. As the ampulla comes into view, the proximity of the common duct must be kept in mind.

A very tense, distended gallbladder may need to be decompressed to expose the hepatoduodenal ligament for safe dissection. This can be accomplished with a trochar attached to suction. The defect in the fundus of the gallbladder is clamped when the trochar is removed.

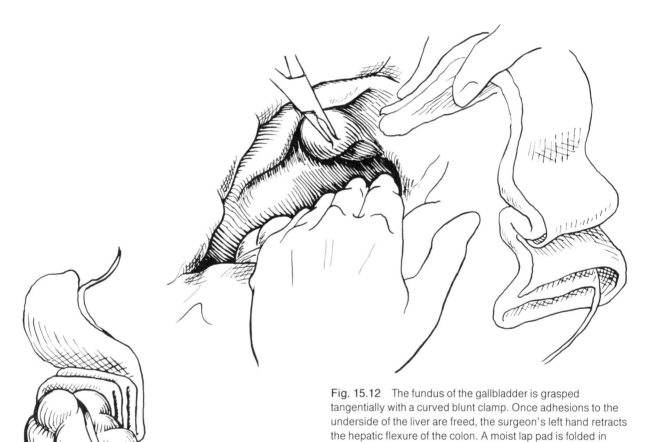

Fig. 15.12   The fundus of the gallbladder is grasped tangentially with a curved blunt clamp. Once adhesions to the underside of the liver are freed, the surgeon's left hand retracts the hepatic flexure of the colon. A moist lap pad is folded in thirds and placed over the left hand down to the fingertips. It is held in place with the right hand while the left is removed.

Fig. 15.13   The remainder of the pad is folded into place accordion fashion. If properly placed, this pad will often hold its position without additional retraction.

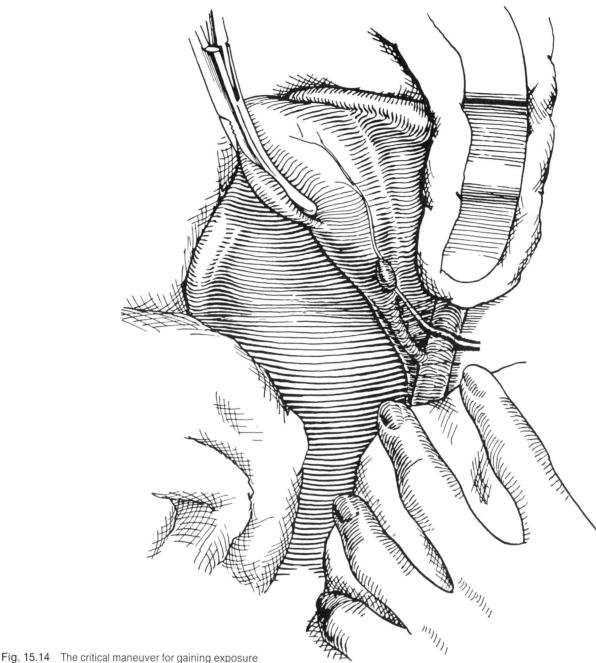

Fig. 15.14   The critical maneuver for gaining exposure involves placing a lap pad and the first assistant's left hand over the duodenum.

The fingers are spread and gently retract duodenum and pancreas toward the midline. This tenses the hepatoduodenal ligament and the fold containing the cystic duct. The index and middle fingertips are placed on either side of the junction between cystic and common duct. Another moist lap pad is held by a narrow Deaver just medial to the gallbladder. An additional clamp may be placed on the ampulla if it is pendulous and obscuring the view of the hepatoduodenal ligament.

The surgeon can now palpate the common duct for stones by placing thumb and index finger on either side of the hepatoduodenal ligament. Any extensive manipulation of the common duct is best done with the surgeon on the patient's left.

The gallbladder should not be palpated yet for fear of forcing stones into the common duct.

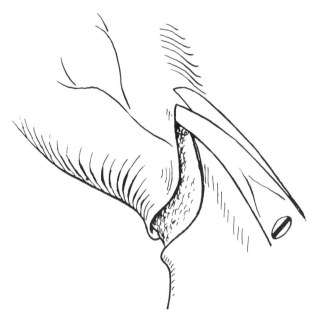

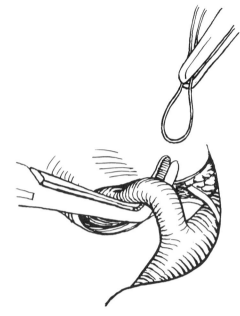

Fig. 15.15 The peritoneum overlying the cystic duct and ampulla is incised as shown. The thickness of the serosal layer can vary tremendously depending on the degree and duration of inflammation. With marked edema the hepatoduodenal ligament can be an inch thick. Under such conditions it may be wise to avoid dissection in this area and settle for a compromise procedure. Options include cholecystostomy or retrograde excision of the gallbladder (leaving a long cystic duct).

Fig. 15.17 The center of a long strand of heavy suture material is passed under the cystic duct.

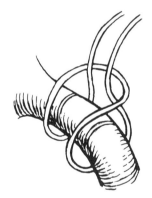

Fig. 15.18 The free ends are brought through the loop, forming a noose that temporarily occludes the duct. This prevents passage of stones during subsequent dissection. It also allows further dissection to confirm that you are indeed around cystic duct and not the common or right hepatic duct. The noose is easily loosened later for the cholangiogram. The true junction with the common duct must be positively identified before the cystic duct is tied.

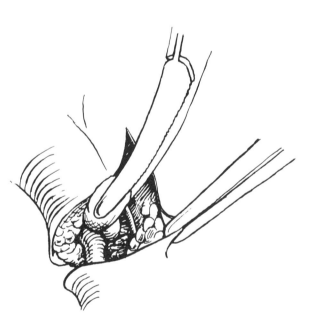

Fig. 15.16 The fat surrounding the cystic duct and artery is gently swept up toward the gallbladder by using a "peanut" sponge. The cystic duct is frequently identified by first finding Calot's node, which overlies it.

There are numerous variations in the anatomy of the cystic duct and cystic artery.

The blood supply to the common duct usually consists of two fine longitudinal vessels lying on either side of the duct in the coronal plane. Dissection of the duct should not be so wide that these vessels are compromised, lest stricture occur secondary to ischemia.

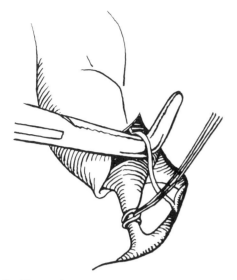

Dissection should clearly demonstrate the cystic artery running onto the body of the gallbladder. A tortuous right hepatic artery can course over the ampulla before turning back into the liver. The dissection will not always look as ideal as in the drawings, but the cleaner the better.

The cystic artery is ligated and divided close to the gallbladder. If the artery escapes, bleeding should be controlled with the Pringle maneuver (compressing the hepatoduodenal ligament), and the vessel should be reclamped under direct vision.

Fig. 15.19 The cystic artery is an end vessel without major anastomoses. When edema and distention compromise the arterial flow, it is the fundus that necroses and perforates. This risk is increased by atherosclerotic changes and diabetic microvascular disease.

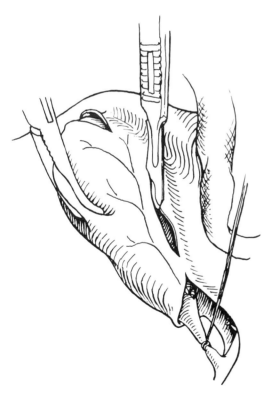

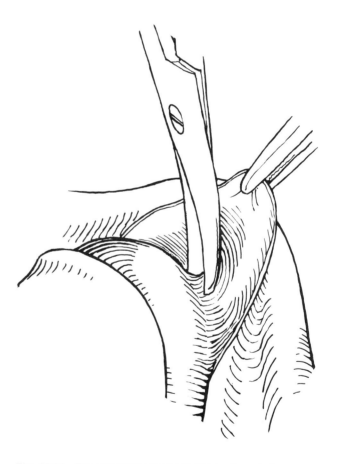

Fig. 15.21 The gallbladder can be excised antegrade from the ampulla; the retrograde dissection is depicted here. With traction on the lip of the peritoneal cuff, the avascular plane between gallbladder and liver is identified. Steady traction is maintained on the gallbladder by increasing the pull as the gallbladder is progessively dissected. The curve of the scissors should follow the gallbladder wall. A single spread followed by a single cut is most efficient.

Fig. 15.20 The peritoneum is incised around the fundus of the gallbladder 1 cm from the liver substance. In some patients the gallbladder is deeply imbedded in liver substance; in others it is almost hanging on a mesentery. A No. 15 blade on a long handle is well suited for this incision. A gentle gliding stroke with the belly of the blade will divide peritoneum without perforating the wall of the gallbladder. This incision is easier if the gallbladder has not been decompressed.

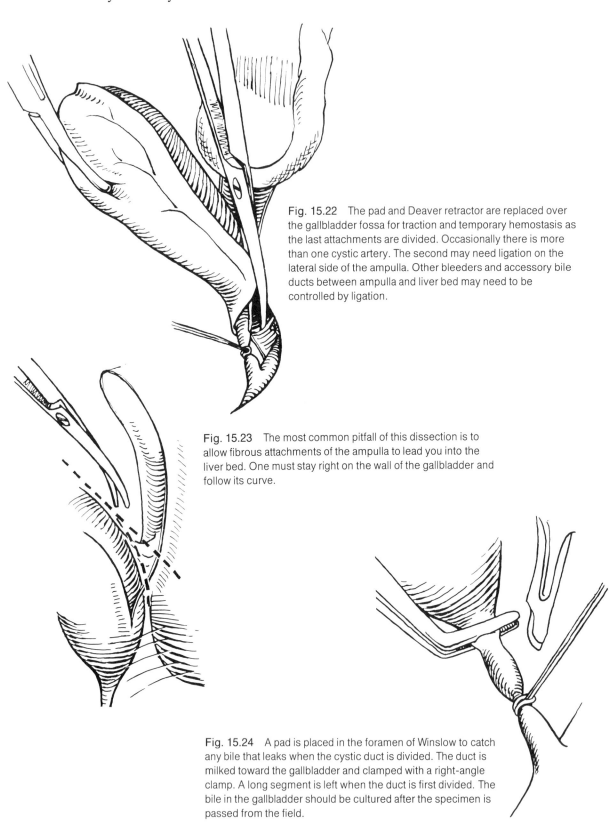

Fig. 15.22   The pad and Deaver retractor are replaced over the gallbladder fossa for traction and temporary hemostasis as the last attachments are divided. Occasionally there is more than one cystic artery. The second may need ligation on the lateral side of the ampulla. Other bleeders and accessory bile ducts between ampulla and liver bed may need to be controlled by ligation.

Fig. 15.23   The most common pitfall of this dissection is to allow fibrous attachments of the ampulla to lead you into the liver bed. One must stay right on the wall of the gallbladder and follow its curve.

Fig. 15.24   A pad is placed in the foramen of Winslow to catch any bile that leaks when the cystic duct is divided. The duct is milked toward the gallbladder and clamped with a right-angle clamp. A long segment is left when the duct is first divided. The bile in the gallbladder should be cultured after the specimen is passed from the field.

A cystic duct cholangiogram should be performed (unless there are major contraindications) because of the unreliability of simple palpation in detecting common duct stones. The study is performed using sterile field technique.

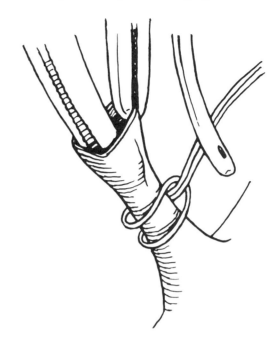

Fig. 15.25 The cut edge of the cystic duct is grasped and the noose is loosened. It may be necessary to dilate the duct with the tips of a fine clamp or a probe. The proper catheter size is selected (usually 14–18 gauge) and the distance to the junction is measured on the catheter.

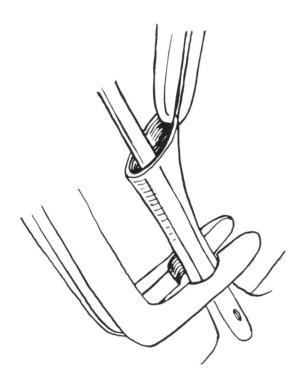

If the catheter is pushed beyond the cystic duct-common duct junction, it can perforate the opposite wall of the common duct. Threading the catheter into the proximal or distal common duct can result in an incomplete cholangiogram. If the cystic duct is too tiny or the valves make it impossible to pass the catheter, a 25-gauge butterfly needle can be used to inject contrast medium directly into the common duct. A cystic duct clamp is shown securing the catheter in position. This is placed to the right side and does not impair radiologic visualization of the duct. The commonly used alternative is to tie the catheter in place.

Fig. 15.26 The catheter is filled with saline and flushed slowly as it is inserted.

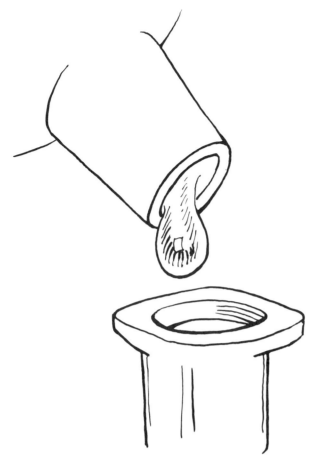

A straight connector is preferable to a three-way stopcock with two syringes because the latter tends to harbor air bubbles, which give false-positive radiologic findings. The syringe should be held upright and tapped to keep air bubbles out of the tip and catheter.

Fig. 15.27   The catheter is aspirated and flushed with saline, and the syringe is disconnected. Before the syringe containing the contrast medium is attached, the connector should be filled to the brim.

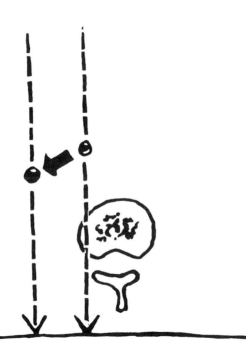

Fig. 15.28   Tilting the patient to his right rotates the common duct off the spine and gives a clearer picture. This can be done by placing bolsters under the patient's left side preoperatively. It can also be accomplished by tilting the whole table to the right. This theoretically puts the grid on the x-ray plate out of alignment with the beam, but in practice it usually results in a sharp, clear picture.

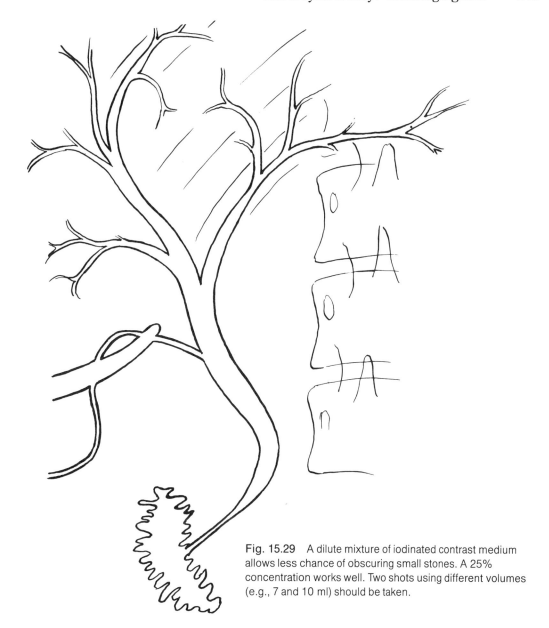

Fig. 15.29   A dilute mixture of iodinated contrast medium allows less chance of obscuring small stones. A 25% concentration works well. Two shots using different volumes (e.g., 7 and 10 ml) should be taken.

The contrast medium should not be injected against great resistance. If easy injection is not possible, check the position of the catheter. High-pressure injection can force contrast medium and infected bile into the pancreatic duct and trigger a postoperative pancreatitis.

A normal cholangiogram shows no filling defects, no sharp cut-off of hepatic radicles, and smooth tapering of the distal common duct. There should be free flow of contrast medium into the duodenum.

While the cholangiogram films are being developed, the gallbladder bed can be checked for hemostasis.

Fig. 15.30   If the x-ray films are normal, the catheter is removed and the duct is ligated close to but not flush with the common duct.

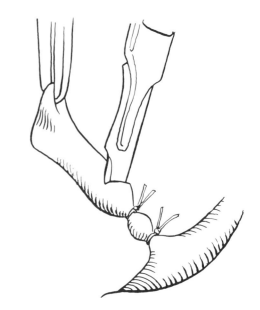

Tenting of the common duct while ligating the cystic duct is a major cause of common duct injury. The x-ray film should demonstrate anomalies such as a long cystic duct sharing a wall with the common duct. The excess cystic duct is excised. A segment of cystic duct sharing a common wall with the common duct should not be disturbed.

The pad in the foramen of Winslow is removed, and the area copiously lavaged with saline.

Fig. 15.31   The gallbladder bed may be left open or closed at the surgeon's discretion.

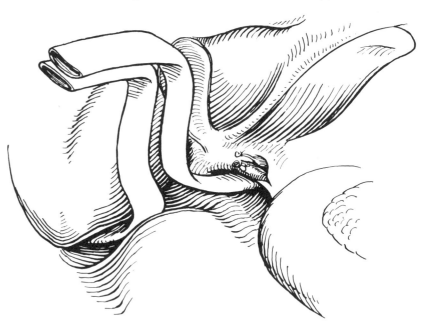

The popularity of not draining after cholecystectomy has waxed and waned over the years. There is ample evidence to support the advocates of not draining a clean dry field. When drainage is elected, two Penrose drains are brought out through a separate stab wound. One may be placed in Morrison's pouch between the kidney and liver, and the other can be located in the foramen of Winslow, or they can both be placed in Morrison's pouch. Their purpose is to allow drainage of bile, blood, or serum that may leak from raw surfaces in the first 24 hours. They are removed separately on the second to fourth day if no evidence of bile leakage is present.

The abdomen is closed by any standard method (see the discussion and depiction of abdominal closure in Chapter 12).

Chapter 16

Small Bowel Resection

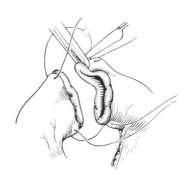

Common surgical pathology of the small bowel includes infarction, trauma, Crohn's disease, Meckel's diverticulum, and polyps. In addition, procedures done for peptic ulcer, and biliary and pancreatic disease use parts of the small bowel for continuity and drainage. Segmental resection of the ileum for traumatic perforation is depicted in the following sequence.

The segment shown in Fig. 16.1 is held up to the light to transilluminate the mesenteric vessels. Defining the vessels in this way may not be possible with the thickened mesentery of Crohn's disease. The site of transsection is chosen to remove all potentially injured bowel at the margins of the wound and to leave a good blood supply to the cut ends. Note that the bowel is supported by the fingertips pinching the mesentery, not the bowel wall. Excessive manipulation of the bowel may prolong postoperative ileus.

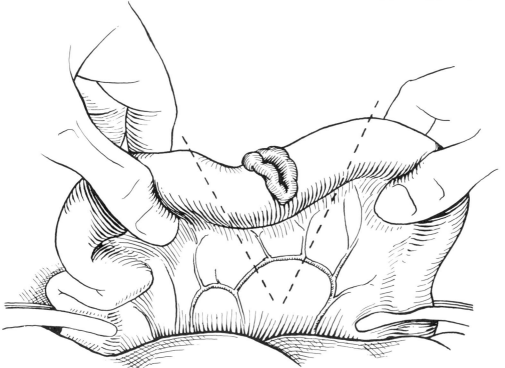

Fig. 16.1 The abdomen has been carefully explored for other injuries. A generous margin of normal bowel is isolated by using atraumatic intestinal clamps. The clamps are placed after bowel contents are milked away from the injured segment. The rest of the field is protected with moist lap pads.

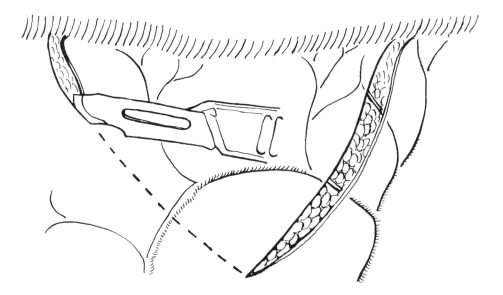

Fig. 16.2   One side of the mesenteric serosa is incised lightly in the shape of a V. This facilitates isolating and precisely ligating the mesenteric vessels.

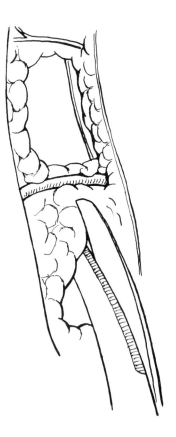

Fig. 16.3   The space between major mesenteric vessels is mostly avascular. With the aid of backlighting, this tissue can be divided right up to the vessels. The vessels can then be precisely clamped, divided, and ligated with a minimum of extraneous tissue.

The alternate method of dividing mesentery uses a series of clamps placed heel-to-toe along the line of division. It is then necessary to mass ligate the tissue in each clamp. Although less desirable, this method may be necessary when the mesentery is thickened and the vessels cannot be individually identified. A vessel that retracts into such a thick mesentery is difficult to control. Injury to adjacent blood vessels may result.

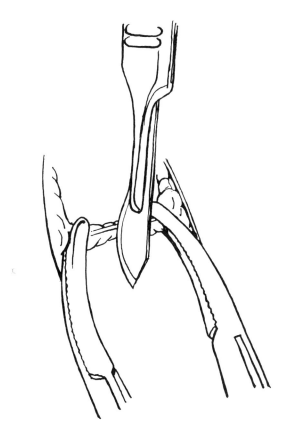

Fig. 16.4   The vessels are sharply divided. Major trunks are doubly ligated or suture ligated.

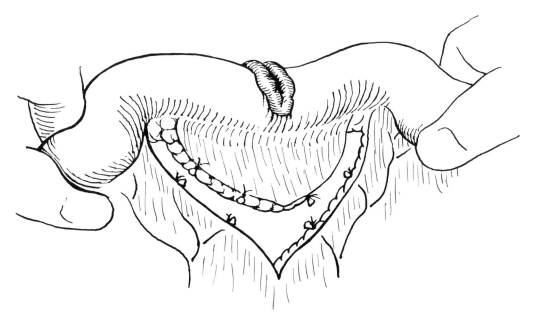

Fig. 16.5   The mesenteric wedge is complete up to the small vessels next to the bowel wall. The shallower this wedge is, the more vessels there are to individually divide. A deep wedge taking a main trunk vessel is quick but compromises the blood supply to the remaining ends. The proper incision lies between the two extremes.

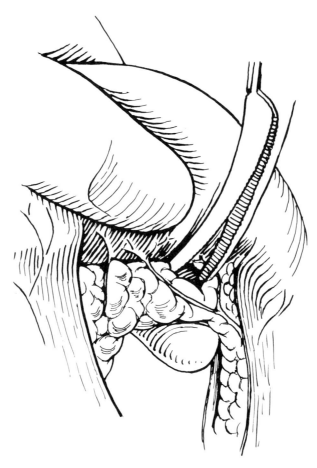

Fig. 16.6   The sites of transsection are prepared by dissecting the small branches adjacent to the bowel.

An index finger pressing up behind the mesenteric border helps define the margin of bowel wall. A mosquito clamp is oriented so that the curve follows the contour of the bowel wall. A space is created between the vessels so that they may be clamped and divided. The distal tie should incorporate a minimal amount of tissue. A bulky wad left on the bowel wall interferes with construction of the anastomosis. A 1 cm cuff of bowel wall usually leaves enough room for suturing without compromising the blood supply to the cut end. Pulsatile vessels should be visible up to the cut edge of the mesentery.

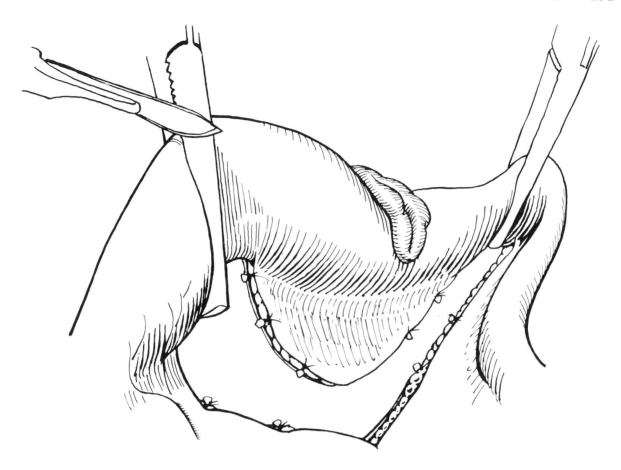

Fig. 16.7 Crushing clamps are placed across the bowel at
the chosen sites. They are angled slightly away from each
other on the antimesenteric border. The antimesenteric corner
is farthest from the blood supply, and this bevel helps ensure
adequate flow from intramural vessels.

The bowel is transsected outside the clamps with a sawing motion of the knife right on the clamp. Suction is kept ready for any residual bowel content. Placing two clamps at each site and cutting between is unnecessary unless there will be a delay before the anastomosis is done. In that case the crushed margin is excised before anastomosis. A sealed division is also accomplished with the gastrointestinal anas-tomosing stapler. The bowel ends are observed for ischemic color change and adequate bleeding at the cut margins. Some submucosal vessels may need to be clamped and ligated with fine (4–0) suture material. If significant bleeders are not controlled, the resulting hematoma may cause obstruction or disruption of the anastomosis.

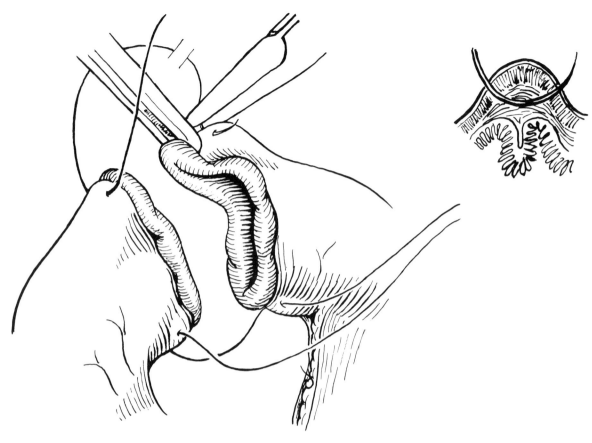

Fig. 16.8   The cut ends should remain together when released, demonstrating that there will be no tension on the suture line. Stay sutures (e.g., 3–0 silk) are placed at the mesenteric and antimesenteric borders.

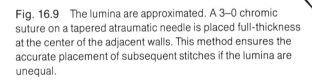

Fig. 16.9   The lumina are approximated. A 3–0 chromic suture on a tapered atraumatic needle is placed full-thickness at the center of the adjacent walls. This method ensures the accurate placement of subsequent stitches if the lumina are unequal.

The needle should enter the bowel perpendicular to the surface and go deep enough to penetrate submucosa before exiting. The submucosa contains most of the collagen in the bowel wall and is therefore the strongest layer. The term "seromuscular stitch" is a misnomer. When a properly placed needle is lifted, compression of submucosal vessels causes blanching on the serosal surface. A shallow tangential bite of muscle will only cut through.

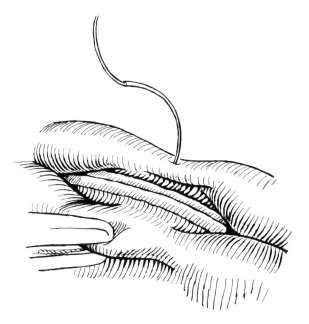

Fig. 16.10   The mucosa at the cut edges becomes progressively more edematous with manipulation.

The ballooning mucosa may be dealt with by the following strategy. The mucosa is gently retracted to expose submucosa and muscularis so that the full-thickness stitch can be placed under direct vision. The entry and exit points are placed a few millimeters from the mucosal edge. Most of the mucosa in any stitch will necrose and slough. Thus, if a large amount of mucosa were included, the stitch would loosen accordingly when the slough occurs. A large amount of mucosa in the anastomosis can also create a temporary obstruction. The knots should be tied so that tissues are just approximated.

Fig. 16.11   The center suture is tied and is run toward one corner as a simple continuous stitch.

Although interrupted sutures decrease the chance of purse-stringing, which creates an undesirably tight diaphragm, the small-bowel lumen is usually wide enough for a careful continuous suture to work well. The continuous suture is also quicker. The absorbable suture material lends additional assurance that a purse-string effect would be only temporary. At the corner the stitches are placed in two bites for accuracy.

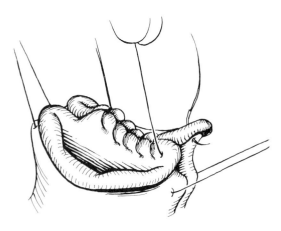

Fig. 16.12   The sutures are placed inside-to-out and outside-to-in until the corner is turned.

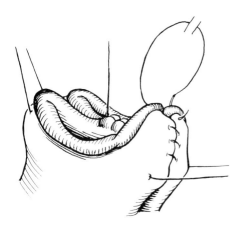

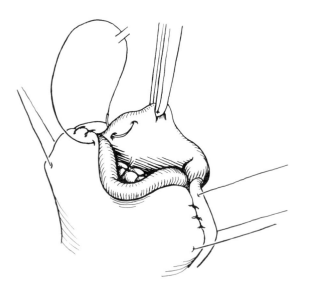

Fig. 16.13   A second chromic suture is placed in the center and tied. The free end is tied to the free end of the first suture. The second suture is run in the opposite direction until that corner is turned. The bowel is oriented so that the surgeon is comfortable, preferably working toward himself. A Connell stitch is then started to complete the anterior suture line.

Fig. 16.14   As each stitch is pulled tight, the opposite bowel wall is gently turned under to invert the mucosa. Remember large bites of mucosa should be avoided by carefully planning where the needle penetrates. If accurate placement is not possible with a single in-and-out passage of the needle, two bites should be used. This is necessary as the opening gets smaller toward the center.

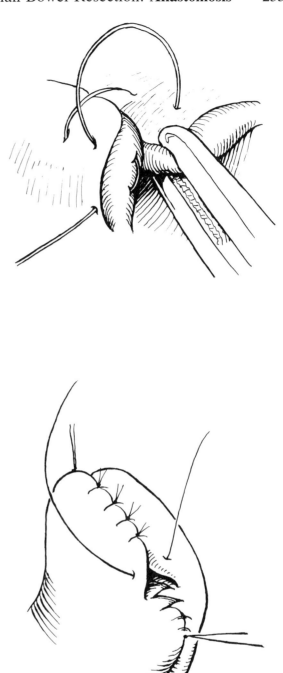

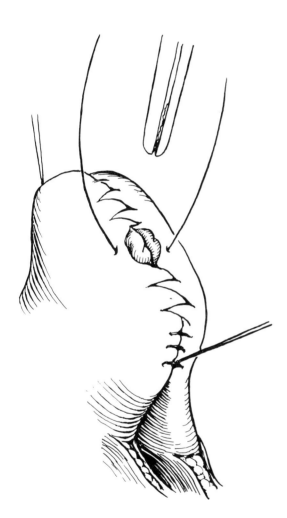

Fig. 16.15   When the two suture ends are opposite each other, the remaining bud of mucosa is carefully invaginated as the ends are tied. The completed Connell inverting suture line looks like a zigzag pattern on the serosal surface. The stay sutures are tied.

Fig. 16.16   An interrupted nonabsorbable 3–0 outer layer is now placed. The stitches again must go deep enough to include submucosa. Do not hestitate to take these stitches in two bites. Vessels should be avoided at the mesenteric border. If a significant vessel is punctured, the safest course is to remove the stitch and apply gentle pressure for a few minutes to prevent a suture-line hematoma. Occasionally, tying the suture will control such a bleeder.

The outer layer on one side may be placed before beginning the inner layer. This approach is useful when suturing a bowel segment that is not mobile enough to flip easily from side to side.

The lumen at the anastomosis may be palpated between two fingers to check for patency.

A horizontal mattress stitch that skims under the serosal leaf may be helpful when the edge is friable. The procedure for an end-to-side and side-to-side anastomosis is very similar to that described above. A continuous outer layer is usually employed for a side-to-side anastomosis.

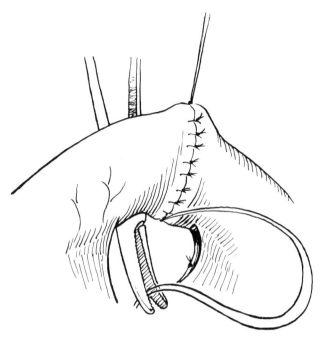

Fig. 16.17 The mesenteric stay suture is passed beneath the bowel and the opposite side of the anastomosis is exposed. The interrupted outer layer is completed on the second side.

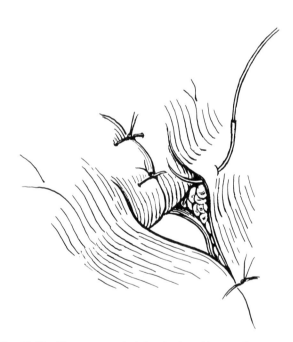

Fig. 16.18 The mesenteric defect is closed by suturing one serosal leaf to its counterpart. Care is taken not to injure the vessels.

The Stapled Bowel Anastomosis

One example of the use of surgical staplers is presented here as an alternate method of small bowel anastomosis. This is called a functional end-to-end anastomosis. The qualification "functional" will be made clear as the method is described. The method shown starts with open bowel ends for simplicity. If the bowel had been transsected using the gastrointestinal anastomosing instrument, each end would be sealed with a double row of staples. In that case the antimesenteric corners would first be cut diagonally with a heavy Mayo scissors to permit introduction of one jaw of the gastrointestinal anastomosing instrument into each lumen. With open lumina the bowel walls are oriented to that the antimesenteric borders are opposed between the jaws (Fig. 16.19).

Firing of the instrument creates a longitudinal opening sealed with double rows of staples (Fig. 16.20). Stay sutures are placed, which help open the new communication so that the inverted staple lines can be inspected for significant bleeding. An additional suture is placed at the distal end of the staple lines on the serosal side to ensure the seal at that junction.

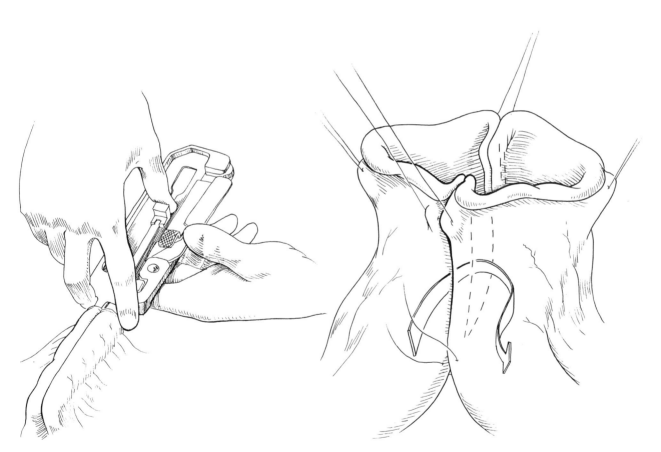

Fig. 16.19 The antimesenteric sides of the bowel ends are stapled and opened with the gastrointestinal anastomosing instrument.

Fig. 16.20 Stay sutures open the lumen so that the stapled edges of the new channel can be inspected for bleeding.

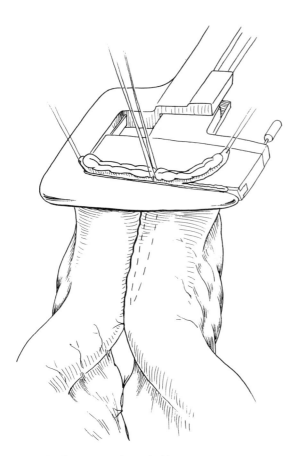

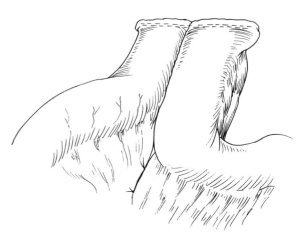

Fig. 16.22   The result is functionally indistinguishable from a hand-sewn end-to-end anastomosis.

Fig. 16.21   The thoracoabdominal instrument closes the bowel ends.

The stay sutures are then used to position the open bowel ends within the jaws of a thoracoabdominal instrument to complete the closure (Fig. 16.21). This may be accomplished with a single long staple line or two intersecting staple lines, depending on the width of the opening. The excess tissue protruding beyond the thoracoabdominal instrument jaws is removed before the jaws are opened. When only the corners of previously closed bowel ends have been opened, as described earlier, one small additional staple line is sufficient. The result is physiologically indistinguishable from an end-to-end anastomosis (Fig. 16.22).

Chapter 17

Vascular Anastomosis

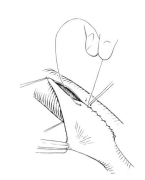

Vascular surgery demands highly refined application of the principles we have been discussing. The surgeon must focus his attention on precise movements and minute details. In few other areas of surgery can momentary loss of concentration produce such disastrous consequences.

Details of technique must be adhered to in an equally rigorous fashion. Asepsis is vital, especially when a synthetic graft is used. If such a graft becomes an infected foreign body, a choice between life and limb often ensues.

Exposure and control are magnified in importance. If proximal and distal control of a major vessel is not securely achieved, exsanguination can occur in minutes.

Tissue handling requires the utmost delicacy. Vascular endothelium is extremely susceptible to injury, which leads to thrombosis. Veins are thin, fragile, and difficult to work with. Sclerotic vessels are hard to sew and tend to crack. Compounding all this, the pressure of the contained blood causes it to leak from any puncture site. This leak is often slow to stop when heparin has been used to prevent clotting in sites distal to the operative occlusion.

Hemostasis is necessary to effectively follow the principles discussed above. Again the interdependence of the basic principles is evident. The synchronous functioning of all these parts can be called good surgical technique.

Technical Points

In performing vascular anastomoses there are a few technical "tricks" that are usually not described in the textbooks of vascular surgery. These technical points contribute to the construction of an easier, quicker, and safer anastomosis.

The routine use of visual magnification in construction of all fine vascular anastomoses allows for the accurate placement of the sutures and the precise identification of the anatomical structures (Fig. 17.1). Surgical loupes of 2.5 to 3.5-power magnification should always be in the armamentarium of the vascular surgeon. They are essential in cases of small anastomoses, endarterectomy of medium size arteries, identification of fine structures such as lymphatic vessels, and in all cases of pediatric vascular surgery.

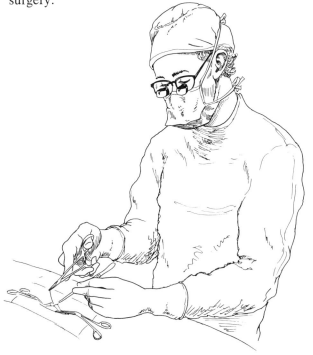

Fig. 17.1 The routine use of visual magnification promotes precise, fine vascular anastomosis.

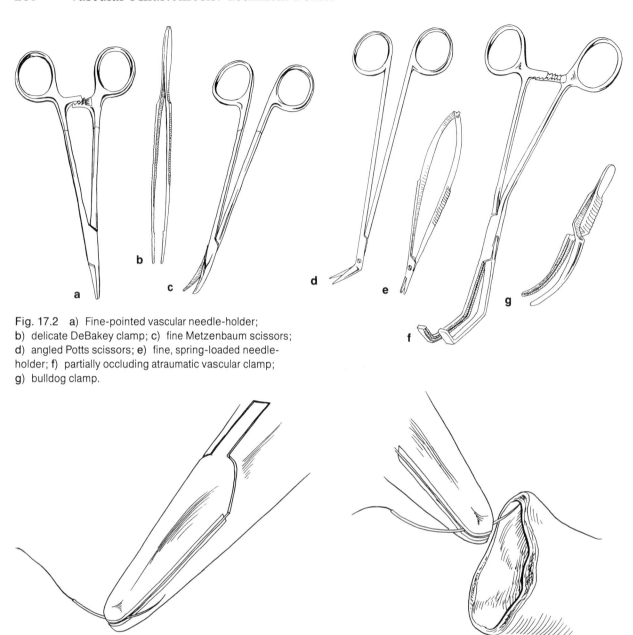

Fig. 17.2   a) Fine-pointed vascular needle-holder;
b) delicate DeBakey clamp; c) fine Metzenbaum scissors;
d) angled Potts scissors; e) fine, spring-loaded needle-
holder; f) partially occluding atraumatic vascular clamp;
g) bulldog clamp.

Fig. 17.3   A fine vascular needle is held at its midpoint by the tip of the needle-holder.

Fig. 17.4   The needle is held closer to the tip to penetrate a calcified vessel wall without bending.

The importance of adequate surgical instruments has been stressed many times. Fine tissue forceps, noncrushing vascular clamps, delicate needle-holders, and a good pair of well-balanced dissecting scissors are the surgeon's jewels (Fig. 17.2). It is not possible to perform a technically good operation without adequate tools. A common mistake is to use a heavy general surgery needle-holder with a fine 5–0 or 6–0 vascular suture. As a result the needle bends or breaks, especially if the vessel is atherosclerotic with a heavily calcified wall. A fine-tipped needle-holder should always be used with such needles, and the tip of the needle-holder should grasp the middle third of the needle (Fig. 17.3). If the needle is held very close to its swaged end, it will frequently bend or break when suturing arterial walls with calcified plaques. In this case the needle should be held very close to its tip, at the junction of its middle and distal thirds (Fig. 17.4).

It is always easier and safer to place the suture from the inside to the outside of the artery, especially when there is severe atherosclerosis. This means that in a graft-to-vessel anastomosis, the suture should enter first the graft from outside to inside and then the patient's artery from inside to outside (Fig. 17.5).

This prevents the detachment of calcified plaques (Fig. 17.6). The suture should always be gently pulled by the first assistant in the same direction in which the needle exited the patient's artery (Fig. 17.7). If the suture is pulled in the opposite direction, the vessel wall will tear (Fig. 17.8).

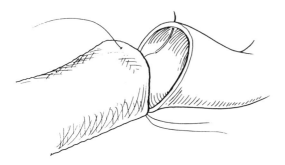

Fig. 17.5   Whenever possible the needle is passed so that it penetrates the patient's vessel from inside to outside.

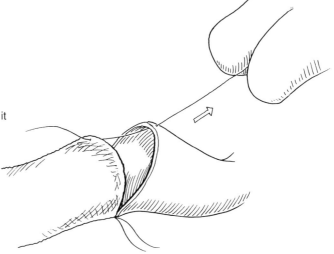

Fig. 17.7   The strand should be pulled through in the direction of penetration.

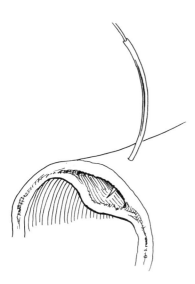

Fig. 17.6   Passing the needle from outside to inside increases the risk of separating calcified plaque and developing a flap.

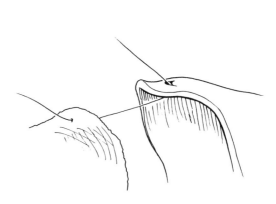

Fig. 17.8   Pulling opposite the direction of penetration widens the suture hole and can tear the vessel.

Considerable time is lost during the construction of a vascular anastomosis by replacing the needle and readjusting its position in the needle-holder after each pass of the suture. To save time the needle should be thrust through the vessel wall until its distal third is visible outside the vessel (Fig. 17.9a). A gentle pull with the fine-tipped needle-holder will expose the middle third of the needle (Fig. 17.9b). At this point the needle-holder is reapplied at the middle third of the needle (Fig. 17.9c), and the pass is completed with the needle already positioned to begin the next cycle.

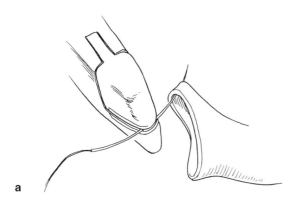

a

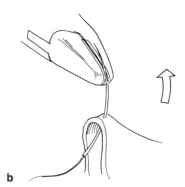

b

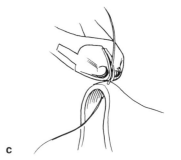

c

Fig. 17.9   a) The needle is passed so that the full distal third is through. b) A gentle pull exposes the middle third. c) The middle third is regrasped, and the needle is in the proper position to start the next cycle.

The following presentation of an end-to-side vein graft to artery anastomosis illustrates the principles of surgical technique. As with all the previous sample procedures the purpose is not to show how to *do* a vascular anastomosis but to show *how* a vascular anastomosis is done.

Arteriotomy

The artery is sharply dissected free from surrounding structures to allow proximal and distal control (Fig. 17.10). Adventitia is not stripped down to bare white arterial wall, since the fine vessels in this layer provide blood supply to the artery. Vascular clamps are placed far enough away to allow adequate working room at either end of the planned arteriotomy. The clamps are tightened only enough to stop blood flow without crushing the vessel wall. A small stab wound is made with a No. 11 blade.

The angled (Potts) vascular scissors opens the arteriotomy to the desired length (Fig. 17.11). The vein graft end may be cut on a bias first and the opening measured against the artery. The alternative is to tailor the bias to fit the arteriotomy. A single smooth cut is made with the scissors to avoid a jagged edge. A fairly long bias provides a gradual transition from the size of the artery to that of the graft. This decreases turbulence that can damage the intima and impede flow.

Stay sutures may be placed at the midpoint of the arteriotomy. It is helpful to include adventitia in this stitch, since it adds strength and prevents the suture from cutting through (Fig. 17.12). A monofilament such as polypropylene is widely favored for vascular work. The size depends on the nature of the vessels, but the basic principle of using the smallest suture possible applies.

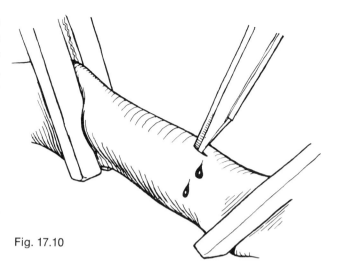

Fig. 17.10

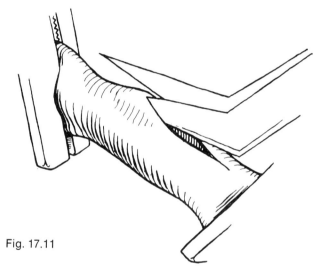

Fig. 17.11

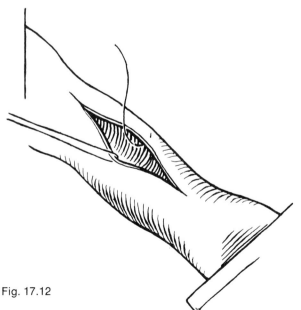

Fig. 17.12

Anchoring Sutures

The reversed vein is cut on an appropriate bias with a single smooth motion of the scissors (Fig. 17.13). Double-armed sutures are placed from inside to out at the heel and toe of the vein and at the corners of the arteriotomy. A smaller bite is taken in the flexible vein than in the artery. Going from inside to out minimizes separation of the intima and subsequent intimal flap dissection.

The assistant holds the vein adventitia with atraumatic vascular forceps and rides the graft down as the heel suture is tied (Fig. 17.14). The free ends are temporarily controlled with rubber-shod clamps, which do not weaken the suture. The proximal suture is then tied as the assistant again relieves tension with his forceps.

One of the suture ends at the heel is passed to the opposite side while the graft is gently elevated (Fig. 17.15). The vessels are moistened frequently with normal saline to prevent injury to the vessel walls from drying.

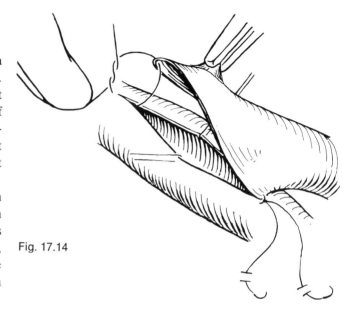

Fig. 17.14

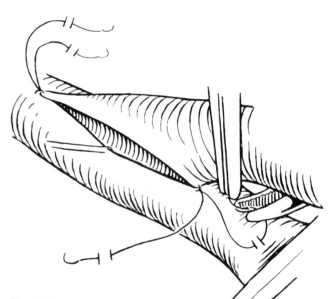

Fig. 17.15

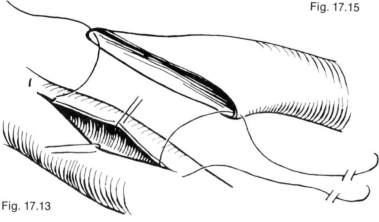

Fig. 17.13

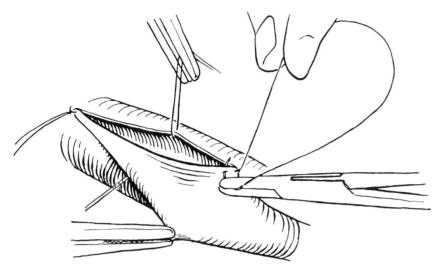

Fig. 17.16   Note the amount of exposure and control shown in this illustration. If this represents the femoral anastomosis of a right femoral-popliteal bypass you are looking from the vantage point of the surgeon. The patient's feet are to your right.

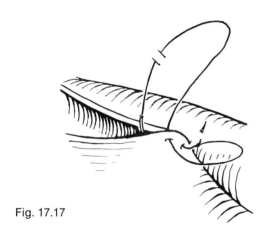

Fig. 17.17

Corner Stitches

The assistant tenses the opposite stay suture with the vascular forceps in his right hand while he follows the surgeon's suture with his left. He will move to release the suture only when the surgeon is ready to take up the slack. The assistant or surgeon will guide the loop to the proper position as it is pulled snug. The surgeon is giving himself countertraction and exposure by holding adventitia with the forceps in his left hand while he passes the suture backhand with his right. The needle is held closer to the point than for other types of suturing, and the motion of passing the needle is close to a straight thrust. Circumstances frequently dictate different patterns of cooperation between surgeon and assistant. Figure 17.16 is just one example.

The corner stitches are taken in two bites for accurate placement and are placed close together initially (Fig. 17.17). The corner presents the greatest danger of leak and is the most difficult spot to correct later. The points of these fine needles are easily bent and should not be grasped with the needle-holders.

The vascular surgeon frequently wears magnifying loupes with a fixed focus. Because the surgeon must keep his eyes focused on the anastomosis, certain unique demands are placed on him, his assistant, and his scrub nurse. He must manipulate his needle with his forceps in the depths of the wound to reseat it in his needle-holder. The assistant must protect the surgeon from obstacles and entanglement in the surrounding field when the surgeon pulls a stitch through and out of his own field of vision. The scrub nurse must have the proper instrument ready in the proper orientation to hand to the surgeon so that the surgeon does not have to look up.

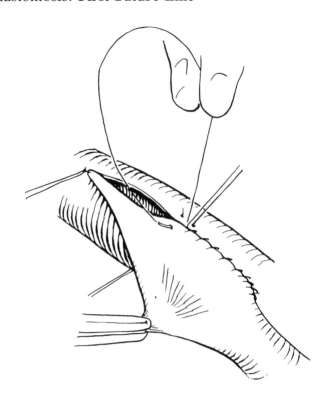

Fig. 17.18

First Suture Line

When the stay suture is reached, it is cut out if it is in the way. The endothelium is the most delicate and vital layer and is protected at all costs. The needle must traverse one endothelium from outside to inside; there is a lesser likelihood of damage in the more flexible vein. With edges lined up accurately, subsequent stitches are placed through both vessel walls at the same time (Fig. 17.18).

Several stitches may be taken with the suture at the toe before the ends are tied together. Close, accurate sutures are also important at the toe. The opposite side is then completed in a similar manner.

Distal clamps are slowly released to expel air before the last stitch is tied. Initial leaks are covered with the gloved finger for a few minutes and usually seal off. Rubber, unlike gauze, will not pull off a clot when removed. Occasionally an additional stitch must be placed.

A concerted application of all the principles of good surgical technique helps ensure a smoothly executed anastomosis. A small break in technique may necessitate redoing an entire anastomosis. The added ischemia time could compromise the survival of a limb.

Epilogue

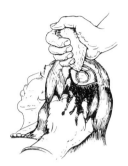

The young doctor enters the emergency room on this, his first day of internship, unaware that on this day 10,000 years before his paleolithic predecessor was straining and sweating with the effort of scraping a hole in his own patient's skull. The intern makes his way over to the patient he was called to see. The patient's head is wrapped with blood-soaked gauze, and as the intern bends closer, the impact of alcohol-saturated breath makes him recoil. He unwinds the gauze, exposing a gaping wound in the parietal area, the edges still actively bleeding. He looks around desperately for help as the patient snores peacefully. A sympathetic nurse notices his plight and comes over carrying gauze and a suture set. She asks if the intern objects to her putting pressure on the wound with gauze while he sets up the suture set and preps. He assures her that he was about to suggest just that. As the intern tries to remember what to do with the paraphernalia on the tray, the ER resident quietly directs a spotlight onto the wound. By the time the intern turns to the wound, the bleeding has almost stopped and the cut is brightly lit and clearly visible. With renewed confidence, the intern proceeds to scrub the wound with prep solution. To his horror the wound begins to bleed more profusely than before. At this point the resident takes pity on him and puts on a pair of gloves. He demonstrates how the bleeding can be controlled by pressing the scalp against the skull on either side of the wound. He offers technical suggestions as the intern sutures the wound and comforting words when the intern forgets how to tie the knots he has practiced a hundred times.

A week later, when the intern sees the patient in clinic, the wound is miraculously healed and free of infection. He knows he has begun to learn important lessons, although he cannot consciously explain exactly what they are. In fact, he has had his first practical lessons in hemostasis, asepsis, exposure, and tissue handling.

A year has passed since that first night in the emergency room. The resident has proven himself reliable and hard working and is about to be rewarded by doing his first cholecystectomy. His chief resident gave him his choice of attending surgeons, and he has chosen one whose clinical and technical skills are respected by all. Standing next to the attending surgeon at the scrub sink, the resident is put at ease by the casual questions put to him. By the end of the scrub, the resident has recited a concise, complete history of the patient's problem and discusses the important surgical considerations. As they enter the operating room, the resident is surprised at the sudden transformation the attending surgeon undergoes. No longer casual and smiling, his face has turned to stone and his manner is cold and precise.

At first the resident is pleased that the attending surgeon remains detached, giving the resident the feeling that he is really in charge of this, his first major abdominal operation. When he finally opens the peritoneum after half an hour of struggling, he suspects something is amiss. It didn't look this hard yesterday when he helped the same attending do a cholecystectomy. After several minutes more of a losing battle to hold the slippery viscera out of the way, the resident looks up despairingly at his attending surgeon, who in a chilling voice says, "OK, now are you ready to do it right?" As the resident vigorously nods his head yes, the attending surgeon spreads his size 8 hand over duodenum and pancreas. Suddenly there is a vast space in the upper abdomen

267

affording a clear view of the anatomy. By the end of the case, the resident has learned, among other things, the importance of proper assistance and how to use that assistance to gain exposure.

The chief resident recalls that first big case as he rides the elevator up to the operating room. On the stretcher next to him is the Chinese seaman he has just examined in the emergency room. A 1 inch steel cable snapped and lashed across the man's abdomen. On examination he has evidence of generalized peritonitis. The man speaks no English, and it is uncertain how long ago he ate. A nasogastric tube has drained a minimal amount of stomach contents. Remembering the subphrenic abscess he saw drained that morning, the complication of a perforated diverticulum, he has started the patient on antibiotics in the emergency room.

He has been given independent privileges and operates without an attending surgeon tonight. He quickly and expertly opens the abdomen through a midline incision – and he groans. The small-bowel lymphatics are whitely engorged with digested fats,

and the abdomen is peppered with grains of rice that continue to pour from a blowout of the proximal ileum. He isolates the perforated segment and lavages the peritoneum with liters of warm saline until he is satisfield that it is clean. He positions his assistants effectively, walls off the damaged bowel, and protects the other exposed viscera with moist pads. Fortunately he has a good scrub nurse with whom he has worked many times. The proper instruments are passed with little verbal exchange. The resident's movements are economical and precise, and his intern marvels at how he completes the procedure so quickly without seeming to rush, while at the same time paying exquisite respect to the tissue he handles.

The chief resident stays to help the new intern put in skin sutures. The intern blushes as he fumbles to tie the knot he has practiced so many times before. The chief resident smiles to himself and begins to teach the intern.

It is our hope that this book will be of help in the beginning.

Appendix:
Summary of Principles

General Principles

I. First do no harm!

II. The surgeon's quality
  A. Behavior pattern
    1. Pay compulsive attention to detail
    2. Make logical decisions
    3. Exercise self-control
    4. Act consistently under stress
    5. Show maturity
    6. Demonstrate leadership
  B. Manual proficiency
    1. Natural dexterity
    2. Practiced skills
    3. Economy of motion
  C. Preparation
    1. Didactic knowledge including anatomy and pathophysiology
    2. Know surgical procedures
    3. Study the patient: operate at the proper time, not too early or too late
    4. Prepare the patient psychologically and physically
    5. Arrangements for surgery
      a) Appropriate assistants
      b) Special instruments
      c) Special studies (e. g., x-ray films)
      d) Consultant support
      e) Post-op facilities (e. g., ICU)
  D. Post-op care: The operation is a brief event in the total care of a patient

III. Asepsis
  A. Follow sterile technique
  B. Avoid environment favorable to bacteria
    1. Do not leave culture media in the wound
      a) Minimize dead tissue
        i) No mass ligature
        ii) Minimal cautery
        iii) Preserve blood supply
        iv) Irrigate to debride mechanically
      b) Minimize blood accumulation by careful hemostasis
      c) Dissect carefully to minimize raw surfaces that ooze serum
      d) Place drains when fluid is likely to collect
    2. Eliminate dead space where culture media accumulate
    3. Minimize foreign material left in the wound
    4. Leave high-risk wounds open to granulate initially
  C. Decrease the inoculum of bacteria present during surgery
    1. Sterilize sources of contamination such as bowel
    2. Work efficiently to decrease exposure time and probability of contamination
    3. Use antibiotics appropriately
      a) Prophylactically when there is high risk of infection
      b) Therapeutically for existing contamination
    4. Dilute bacteria to extinction by copious irrigation
    5. Minimize movement and talking in the operating room
  D. Host resistance should be at normal levels; correct pre-op metabolic, nutritional, and drug-induced problems

IV. Tissue handling
  A. Manipulations
    1. Gentle
    2. Clean, decisive movements
    3. Approximate tissue, do not strangulate it with sutures
    4. Use proper instruments
    5. No mass ligature
  B. Dissection
    1. Sharp
    2. Follow anatomic planes
    3. Preserve functional tissue and keep blood supply intact

4. Mobilize only what is necessary
5. Cut only what can be seen
C. Protect tissue
  1. Keep it moist
  2. Minimize exposure time
  3. Minimize electrocoagulation

V. Hemostasis
  A. Include screening for coagulation defects in pre-op evaluation
  B. Ensure ties
    1. Square knots
    2. The proper number of knots for the material
    3. Suture or double ligation of high-risk vessels
  C. Coagulate precisely to prevent damage to surrounding tissues
  D. Use appropriate clamps to hold vessels securely without injuring adjacent tissue
    1. Grasp the minimal tissue necessary
    2. Choose the correct size clamp for the job
  E. Secure proximal control of major vessels first

VI. Exposure
  A. Positions
    1. Patient
    2. Surgeon
    3. Assistants
  B. Focus and readjust light as the operative field changes
  C. Incision
    1. Make it large enough to allow visibility and maneuverability
    2. Take into account anatomic obstacles when placing it
  D. Retraction is a key to exposure; an adequate incision allows gentle retraction that does not damage tissue
  E. The length of instruments must reflect the depth of the structure on which they are used; they should keep hands out of the line of vision

Wound Healing

I. Factors affecting healing
  A. Infection
    1. Large inoculum of bacteria
    2. Necrotic tissue
    3. Foreign body in the wound

4. Decreased host defense
5. Compromised circulation limiting delivery of defensive elements
B. Compromised circulation
  1. Macrovascular disease
    a) Atherosclerosis
    b) Venous stasis
  2. Compromised microcirculation
    a) Diabetic microvascular disease
    b) Vasculitis
    c) Radiation endarteritis
    d) Strangulating sutures
    e) Pressure dressing
  3. Systematic factors
    a) Anemia
    b) Hypovolemia
    c) Low O_2 tension
    d) Sludging (from hypovolemia, low flow states, hypothermia)
    e) Disseminated intravascular coagulation
C. Circumstances of the wound
  1. Etiology of the wound
  2. Delay of treatment
  3. Age and health of the patient (e.g., chronic debilitating disease)
D. Nutrition
  1. Protein anabolism/catabolism
  2. Effect on host immune competence
  3. Vitamin and mineral cofactors
E. Drugs
  1. Steroids
  2. Anti-inflammatory agents
  3. Cytotoxic drugs
F. Specific agents
  1. Proline analogues inhibit collagen helix formation
  2. β-APN and D-penicillamine inhibit cross-linking

II. Practical considerations
  A. Monitor and treat fluid, electrolyte, and ventilatory derangements to avoid irreversible damage to the microcirculation and cell death
  B. Use good surgical technique (as outlined under General Principles)
  C. Provide nutritional support; parenteral alimentation when needed
  D. Correct local and systemic conditions (above) that adversely affect healing
  E. Replace sutures (or clips) early with paper tape to reduce cross-hatching

F. Technique
1. Incision
   a. Cut along skin lines
   b. Cut between neurovascular structures
   c. Follow flexion creases
2. Wounds
   a. Debride until only healthy tissue remains
   b. Leave contaminated wounds open
   c. Skin graft indurated wounds

Surgical Knots and Suture Materials

I. Hand ties
A. Choose a throw compatible with the initial position of the working strand
B. Work toward and away from your body
C. Finish with the working strand on the side opposite to which it started
D. Position your body comfortably
E. Grasp a comfortable length of the strands so that the index finger just reaches the knot
F. Set up a loose, even loop
G. Pass the working strand cleanly through the loop
H. Maintain equal tension on each strand to keep an open round loop until the throw is set
I. Place the tightening finger down on the strand that is dependent to (below) the knot
J. Tighten strands in a straight line with the knot
K. Approximate tissue, do not strangulate it
L. Tighten the knot with a final jiggle on the strand
M. Alternate throws to form a square knot
N. The number of throws necessary for a secure knot depends on the suture material

II. Instrument ties
A. Leave the working end short
B. Place the needle holder between the strands
C. Loop the long end over the needle holder
D. Grasp the end of the working strand
E. Pull the strands toward the side opposite to which they started
F. Maintain equal tension and an open loop
G. Alternate directions for a square knot

III. Suture materials
A. Knot security
1. Accuracy of tying
2. Type of knot
   a) Flat throws are essential
   b) A half hitch is a slip knot; it has no holding power
   c) Security is generally improved by additional throws
3. Tensile strength
   a) High tensile strength allows the use of finer material, which leaves less foreign body in the wound
   b) Breakage is inversely proportional to tensile strength and diameter
4. Coefficient of friction
   a) High coefficient of friction allows fewer throws for a smaller secure knot, which leaves less foreign body in the wound
   b) Slippage is a function of the coefficient of friction and the accuracy with which the knot was tied
   c) Slippage occurs at a much lower strain level than breakage
   d) A high coefficient of friction causes more tissue trauma as the suture is pulled through
   e) Braided materials have a higher coefficient of friction than monofilaments
B. Absorbable suture materials
1. Natural (catgut)
   a) Plain
      i) Rapid absorption ($\sim$ 10 days)
      ii) Marked tissue reaction
   b) Chromic
      i) Surface hardened with chromic acid
      ii) Slower absorption ($\sim$ 21 days)
      iii) Less tissue reaction
   c) Marked decrease in knot security and tensile strength when wet; tails must be left long
2. Synthetic absorbable materials (polyglycolic acid, polyglactin 910, polydioxanone)
   a) Polyglycolic acid and polyglactin 910 are braided; higher coefficient of friction than catgut
   b) Less tissue reaction than catgut
   c) Lose strength by 21 days
3. Mandatory use where nonabsorbable materials stimulate stone formation
   a) Biliary tract
   b) Genitourinary tract

C. Nonabsorbable suture materials
  1. Silk
    a) Excellent handling characteristics
    b) Average knot-holding ability and tensile strength
    c) Like all braided materials, has interstices that may harbor bacteria
  2. Dacron polyester
    a) Strongest nonabsorbable material except wire
    b) Excellent knot security
    c) Disadvantages of braided materials (friction, interstices)
    d) Does not handle as well as silk
    e) Coating decreases both drag and knot security
  3. Monofilament plastics (nylon, polypropylene, polyethylene, polybutester)
    a) Nonreactive
    b) Slide easily through tissue
    c) Intermediate tensile strength
    d) Fair to poor knot security; require several flat throws
    e) Stiff, handle poorly
  4. Polytetrafluoroethylene: a hybrid material with flexibility, strength and compressibility
  5. Stainless steel wire
    a) Strongest
    b) Nonreactive
    c) Most secure material when knotted (twisted wires have negligible security)
    d) Hardest to manipulate
  6. Mandatory use when long-term holding power is necessary, as in vascular anastomosis

Instruments

I. Categories of instruments
  A. Cutting
  B. Grasping
    1. Traumatic
    2. Atraumatic
  C. Retractors
    1. Manual
    2. Self-retaining

II. Basic principle: Choose the instrument of the proper size and strength for the job

Basic Surgical Maneuvers

I. Cutting
  A. Scalpel
    1. Attach and detach blade using a clamp
    2. Hold with a balanced, relaxed grip
    3. Efficient motion displaces a minimum number of joints
    4. Fine dissection involves only interphalangeal joint movement; the heel of the hand is stabilized on the skin
    5. Keep the blade perpendicular to the cut structure
    6. Sharp dissection is least traumatic
  B. Scissors
    1. Most effective when kept in the axis of the forearm
    2. Right to left is the most efficient direction for use
    3. The points may face the dorsal or volar surface of the hand to achieve a full 360° rotational range
    4. A pronated position gives finer control
    5. Dissect with a single spread followed by a single cut
    6. Make fine cuts with the tips of the scissors, gross cuts with the heel
    7. Brace the wrist holding the suture scissors on the other arm; hold the suture out of the cutter's line of vision
    8. Tense structures to cut cleanly and easily
    9. Orient the curve of the scissors to follow the plane of the structure
    10. Cut one layer at a time

II. Grasping
  A. Forceps
    1. Use for manipulation and fine traction
    2. Hold with a gentle, balanced grip
    3. Toothed forceps concentrate forces on a small amount of tissue and give maximal holding power with minimal tissue destruction
    4. Use special multitoothed forceps for delicate tissue
    5. Grasp only the adventitial support of delicate structures (blood vessels, nerves, ducts)
    6. Hold the tissue immediately adjacent to where a stitch is being placed; do not release until the needle is withdrawn

B. Clamps
1. Limit blunt dissection to loose areolar tissue
2. Isolate a length of tissue adequate to clamp securely, leaving room to cut between clamps, tie the ends, or regrasp if an end escapes
3. Clamp with the tips, leaving a small overhang to tie around
4. Leave a slightly longer stump on the business end of a vessel
5. Tie around the most superficial clamp first

C. Tying
1. Do not pull on a clamped structure
2. Elevate the rings to pass a ligature; lower the rings and raise the points for tying
3. Tie parallel to and immediately below the clamp
4. Release the clamp slowly as the first throw is tightened
5. Flash (partially open and reclose) the clamp when a second tie or suture ligature is needed
6. Learn to release a clamp with either hand
7. Place ligature in the tip of a clamp and hold tense for passing

III. Suturing
A. The needle-holder
1. Traditional grip is with thumb and ring finger in the rings
2. Removing the thumb from the ring allows an improved axis of rotation
3. Hold the needle two thirds of the distance from the point for general purposes
4. Place and pass the needle once only
5. Release the needle when the needle holder is stopped by tissue

B. Suture patterns
1. Make the distance between stitches equal to the width of each stitch
2. The ideal profile of skin sutures is close to a square or rectangle
3. Tie sutures loosely to allow for edema
4. Simple sutures work best in firm tissue
5. The vertical mattress provides precise edge approximation
6. The horizontal mattress achieves eversion
7. The subcuticular suture avoids skin suture marks
8. Make skin suture bites of equal depth and equal distance on each side

9. A tight continuous suture can cause a purse-string constriction
10. Untwist the remaining strand of a continuous suture after several bites
11. A continuous locking suture prevents slippage and aids hemostasis but may strangulate tissue
12. The Connell stitch is a continuous inverting suture commonly used for the inner layer of bowel anastomoses
13. The Lembert stitch is used for the outer layer of bowel anastomoses; its strength depends on inclusion of the submucosal layer
14. The Halsted stitch is an interrupted seromuscular horizontal mattress; the Cushing stitch is continuous

IV. Hemostasis
A. Delay dealing with multiple small bleeders by pressing with lap pads; many will stop
B. Glove rubber will not pull off a formed clot when used to stop a small bleeder; gauze will
C. Release temporary pressure only when ready to deal with the bleeder
D. Press against a hard underlying structure when it is available
E. Tent up a membranous structure to expose and control a bleeder within that structure
F. Control mesenteric bleeders by pinching on either side of the mesentery
G. To clamp bleeders in the subdermal plexus, point the clamp tip up toward the dermis
H. Evert the sides of the wound at the end of the procedure to expose any remaining bleeding points
I. Suture-ligate major vessels
J. Use small individual sutures for the ends of large vessels
K. Use the least amount of the finest appropriate suture material to leave minimal foreign body in the wound
L. Electrocoagulation
1. Make sure only the tip of the clamp is touching tissue
2. Pinch the clamped tissue with gauze to remove blood
3. Clamp a minimum amount of tissue
4. Apply the electrosurgical tip to any accessible part of the clamp
5. Turn current off as soon as the effect is achieved

6. Use forceps in place of clamps for rapid coagulation of multiple small bleeding points
7. Direct application of the tip causes carbon buildup that must be scraped off
8. Do not wipe the coagulum off; dab if necessary

III. Retraction
 A. The human hand is the best retractor
 B. Choose a retractor of the proper size and shape
 C. Use moist pads to insulate tissue from metal
 D. Always retract gently
  1. Excessive, prolonged pressure damages tissue
  2. If excessive traction is necessary for exposure, the incision is too small
 E. Hand-held retractors
  1. Advantages
   a) Continuous control
   b) Precise adjustments
   c) Assistant can relax tension at appropriate moments
  2. Disadvantages
   a) Fatigue
   b) Poor control if the assistant cannot see the end of the retractor
 F. Self-retaining retractors
  1. Advantages
   a) Maintains a fixed position
   b) Frees assistants for other tasks
  2. Disadvantages
   a) Adjustment takes time and interrupts the flow of the procedure
   b) Does not allow periodic relief of tissue
   c) Bulky

The Surgical Assistant

I. The best assistant is a good surgeon
II. Primary-level assisting
 A. Mechanical and tedious
 B. Should be rewarded with teaching and minor technical jobs
 C. Move only when asked
 D. The surgeon must allow for periods of rest at appropriate intervals
 E. Be aware of the delicacy of the retracted tissues

 F. Should be able to visualize the exposure in order to maintain the proper position

III. Advanced Assisting
 A. Follow the surgeon's lead
 B. Anticipate the next move and respond to the surgeon's cue
 C. Only one hand should be moving in the operative field
 D. Don't abandon one task to do another
 E. Keep out of the surgeon's way

IV. Assisting as an instructor
 A. Remain flexible in response to the level of the resident
 B. The first responsibility is to protect the patient
 C. Anticipate and avoid conflicts in the operating room

The Operating Room Team

I. The Surgeon
 A. Maintains direct communication with all team members and coordinates the team's actions
 B. Responsible for everything that happens in the operating room

II. The Anesthesiologist
 A. Preoperative evaluation of the patient includes careful consideration of airway and systemic problems
 B. Must communicate with the surgeon as the case progresses

III. The Circulator
 A. Provides support for anesthesiologist, surgeon, and scrub nurse
 B. Responsible for patient movement and preparation
 C. Monitors for breaks in sterility
 D. Is in the operating room and available most of the time
 E. Anticipates equipment needs
 F. Monitors and reports blood loss
 G. Helps keep count of needles and sponges
 H. Must accurately label and dispatch specimens

IV. The Scrub Nurse
 A. Provides surgical tools and guards the sterile field

B. Always maintains attention on the operative field
C. Anticipates needs
D. Stands in a position from which instruments can be passed easily
E. Places instruments accurately in hand

F. Chooses instruments of proper length
G. Identifies the drug and dose when medications are passed to the surgeon

V. The interaction of surgical team members is, ideally, calm and professional

Selected References

Introduction

Cruse, P. J. E. Preparing the patient for operation. *Bulletin, American College of Surgeons* May 1981.

Beck, W. C. Operating room illumination: The current state of the art. *Bulletin, American College of Surgeons* May 1981.

History of Surgical Technique

Majno, G. *The Healing Hand: Man and Wound in the Ancient World.* Cambridge: Harvard University Press, 1975.

Burket, W. C. (ed.) *Surgical Papers by William Stewart Halsted.* Baltimore: The Johns Hopkins Press, 1924 (third printing 1961).

Wagensteen, O. H., and Wagensteen, S. D. University *The Rise of Surgery, from Empiric Craft to Scientific Discipline.* Minneapolis: University of Minnesota Press, 1979.

Ancient Surgical Instruments

Milne, J. S. *Surgical Instruments in Greek and Roman Times.* New York: Augustus M. Kelley, 1970.

Wound Healing

Peacock, E. E., and VanWinkle, W. *Wound Repair.* Philadelphia: W. B. Saunders Company, 1984.

Hunt, T. K., and Dunphy, J. E. *Fundamentals of Wound Management,* New York: Appleton-Century-Crofts, 1980.

Surgical Knots and Suture Materials

Tera, H., and Aberg, C. Tensile strengths of twelve types of knot employed in surgery, using different suture materials. *Acta Chirurgica Scand.* 142:1 (1976).

Surgical Needles

Trier, W. C. Considerations in the choice of surgical needles. *Surgery, Gynecology and Obstetrics* 149:84 (1979).

Surgical Drains

Moss, J. P. Historical and current perspectives on surgical drainage. *Surgery, Gynecology and Obstetrics* 152:517 (1981).

Yates, J. L. An experimental study of the local effects of peritoneal drainage. *Surgery, Gynecology and Obstetrics,* 1:473 (1905).

The Operating-Room Team

Atkinson, L. J., and Kohn. M. L. *Berry and Kohn's Introduction to Operating Room Technique.* New York: McGraw-Hill Book Company, 1986.

Surgical Staplers

Steichen, F. M., and Ravitch, M. M., *Stapling in Surgery.* Chicago: Year Book Medical Publishers, 1984.

Microsurgery

Gibson, T. Early free grafting: The restitution of parts completely separated from the body. *British Journal of Plastic Surgery* 18:1 (1965).

Serafin, D., and Buncke, H. *Microsurgical Composite Tissue Transplantation.* St. Louis: C. V. Mosby Company, 1979.

Historical Anatomical Works

O'Malley, C. D., and Saunders, J. B. de C. M. *Leonardo da Vinci on the Human Body.* New York: Outlet Book Company, 1983.

Saunders, J. B. de C. M., and O'Malley, C. D. *The Illustrations from the Works of Andreas Vesalius of Brussels.* Cleveland: The World Publishing Company, 1950. Reprinted by Dover Publications, New York, 1913.

Hale, R. B., and Coyle, T. *Albinus on Anatomy.* New York: Watson-Guptil, 1979.

General Anatomy

Williams, P. L., and Warwick, R. *Gray's Anatomy,* 36th British edition. Philadelphia: W. B. Saunders Company, 1980.

Clemente, C. D. *Anatomy: A Regional Atlas of the Human Body.* Baltimore-Munich: Urban & Schwarzenberg, 1987.

Surgical Anatomy

Anson, B. J., and McVay, C. B. *Surgical Anatomy.* Philadelphia: W. B. Saunders Company, 1984.

Thorek, P. *Anatomy in Surgery.* Philadelphia: J. B. Lippincott, 1985.

General Surgery

Texts

Sabiston, D. C., Jr. (ed.) *Davis-Christopher Textbook of Surgery, The Biological Basis of Modern Surgical Practice.* Philadelphia: W. B. Saunders Company, 1981.

Schwartz, S. I. (ed.) *Principles of Surgery.* New York: McGraw-Hill Book Company, 1983.

Atlases

Zollinger, R. M., and Zollinger, R. M., Jr. *Atlas of Surgical Operations.* New York: Macmillan Publishing Company, 1975.

Madden, J. L., *Atlas of Technics in Surgery.* New York: Appleton-Century-Crofts, 1964.

Minor Procedures

Grabb, W. C., and Smith, J. W. *Plastic Surgery, A Concise Guide to Clinical Practice.* Boston: Little, Brown and Company, 1980.

Vander Salm, T. J. *Atlas of Bedside Procedures.* Boston: Little, Brown and Company, 1979.

Hernia

Nyhus, L. M., and Condon, R. E., *Hernia.* Philadelphia: J. B. Lippincott, 1978.

Gastrointestinal Surgery

Goligher, J. C. *Surgery of the Anus, Rectum and Colon.* London: Balliere Tindall, 1983.

Vascular Surgery

Rutherford, R. *Vascular Surgery.* Philadelphia: W. B. Saunders Co., 1984.

Cooley D., and Wukasch, C. *Techniques in Vascular Surgery.* Philadelphia: W. B. Saunders Co., 1979.

Index